Keto Vegan

2 Books in 1: Keto Vegan Cookbook for Beginners & Keto for Women over 50, A Gentler Approach to Ketogenic, Plant-Based Diet for an Effective Weight Loss and Staying Healthy After 50

Thomas Slow

Text Copyright © Thomas Slow

All rights reserved. No part of this guide may be reproduced in any form without permission in writing from the publisher except in the case of brief quotations embodied in critical articles or reviews.

Legal & Disclaimer

The information contained in this book and its contents is not designed to replace or take the place of any form of medical or professional advice; and is not meant to replace the need for independent medical, financial, legal or other professional advice or services, as may be required. The content and information in this book have been provided for educational and entertainment purposes only.

The content and information contained in this book have been compiled from sources deemed reliable, and it is accurate to the best of the Author's knowledge, information, and belief. However, the author cannot guarantee its accuracy and validity and cannot be held liable for any errors and/or omissions. Further, changes are periodically made to this book as and when needed. Where appropriate and/or necessary, you must consult a professional (including but not limited to your doctor, attorney, financial advisor or such other professional advisor) before using any of the suggested remedies, techniques, or information in this book.

Upon using the contents and information contained in this book, you agree to hold harmless the Author from and against any damages, costs, and expenses, including any legal fees potentially resulting from the application of any of the information provided by this book. This disclaimer applies to any loss, damages or injury caused by the use and application, whether directly or indirectly, of any advice or information presented, whether for breach of contract, tort, negligence, personal injury, criminal intent, or under any other cause of action.

You agree to accept all risks of using the information presented inside this book.

You agree that by continuing to read this book, where appropriate and/or necessary, you shall consult a professional (including but not limited to your doctor, attorney, or financial advisor or such other advisor as needed) before using any of the suggested remedies, techniques, or information in this book.

Table of Contents

Book 1

Table of Contents 3
Introduction 13
Chapter 1: Veganism 15
Chapter 2: Ketogenic Diet 19
Chapter 3: Keto-Vegan Diet 22
Chapter 4: Breakfast Choices 24
    Strawberry Porridge 24
    Gingerbread Porridge 26
    Overnight Strawberry Cheesecake Porridge 27
    Blueberry Quinoa Porridge 28
    Blueberry Chia Pudding 29
    Almond Flour Muffins 30
    Bulletproof Tea 32
    Bulletproof Coffee 33
    Coconut Pancakes 34
    Flaxseed Pancakes 36
    Berry and Nut Cereal 37
    Peanut Butter Fudgy Brownies 38
    Vanilla Golden Turmeric Cereal 40
    Fudge Oatmeal 41
    Raspberry Almond Smoothie 42

Vanilla Overnight Oats 43

Cinnamon Overnight Oats 44

Pumpkin Spice Overnight Oats 45

Smoothie Bowl 46

Eggy Surprise Scramble 47

Bagels 49

Cinnamon Roll Muffins 50

Chapter 5: Lunch & Dinner Favorites **52**

Mushroom Steak 52

Spicy Grilled Tofu Steak 54

Piquillo Salsa Verde Steak 55

Butternut Squash Steak 57

Cauliflower Steak Kicking Corn 59

Pistachio Watermelon Steak 61

BBQ Ribs 62

Spicy Veggie Steaks With veggies 65

Tofu Seitan 68

Stuffed Zucchini 70

Roasted Butternut Squash With Chimichurri 72

Eggplant Pizza 74

Green Avocado Carbonara 76

Curried Tofu 77

Sesame Tofu and Eggplant 78

Tempeh Coconut Curry 80

Tempeh Tikka Masala 82

Caprice Casserole 84

Cheesy Brussel Sprout Bake 86

Tofu Noodle Bowl 88

Cashew Siam Salad 90

Cucumber Edamame Salad 92

Caesar Vegan Salad 93

Mushroom Lettuce Wraps 96

Chapter 6: Side Dishes & Snacks 98

Mixed Seed Crackers 98

Crispy Squash Chips 100

Paprika Nuts 101

Basil Zoodles and Olives 102

Roasted Beetroot Noodles 104

Turnip Fries 105

Lime and Chili Carrots Noodles 107

Pesto Zucchini Noodles 108

Cabbage Slaw 109

Zucchini Chips 110

Peanut Tofu Wrap 112

Cinnamon Granola 113

Chocolate Granola 115

Radish Chips 116

Asparagus Fries 117

Chapter 7: Sauces & Dips 119

Keto-Vegan Ketchup 119

Avocado Hummus 121

Guacamole 122

Keto-Vegan Mayo 123

Peanut Sauce 125

Pistachio Dip 126

Smokey Tomato Jam 127

Tasty Ranch Dressing/Dip 128

Chapter 8: Soups 130

Goulash Soup 130

Celery Dill Soup 132

Broccoli Fennel Soup 133

Broccoli and Cauliflower Soup 135

Keto-Vegan Chili 137

Creamy Avocado Soup 139

Red Onion Soup 140

Thai Pumpkin Soup 141

Zucchini Basil Soup 142

Chapter 9: Smoothies 143

Chocolate Smoothie 143

Chocolate Mint Smoothie 144

Cinnamon Roll Smoothie 145

Coconut Smoothie 146

Maca Almond Smoothie 147

Blueberry Smoothie 148

Nutty Protein Shake 149

Cinnamon Pear Smoothie 150

Vanilla Milkshake 151

Raspberry Protein Shake 152

    Raspberry Almond Smoothie 153

Chapter 10: Desserts **154**

    Keto Chocolate Brownies 154

    Chocolate Fat Bomb 156

    Vanilla Cheesecake 157

    Chocolate Mousse 158

    Avocado Chocolate Mousse 160

    Coconut Fat Bombs 161

    Coconut Cupcakes 162

    Pumpkin Truffles 163

    Raspberry Truffles 164

    Strawberry Ice Cream 166

    Pistachio Gelato 168

    Chocolate Chip Ice Cream 169

    Cinnamon Vanilla Bites 171

    Berry Bites 173

    Coconut Chocolate Balls 174

    Espresso Cups 176

Conclusion **177**
Index for the Recipes **178**

Book 2

Introduction **184**
Chapter 1: Keto – An Overview **186**
    What is the Keto Diet? 186
    What is Ketosis? 188
    How is Insulin Affected by the Keto Diet? 189
    Positive Effects of the Keto Diet 191
    Negative Effects of Keto 192
    Keto Mistakes 194

Chapter 2: Keto for Women Over 50 .... **196**
    General Nutritional Needs for Women Over 50 196
    Gentler Approach to Keto for Women Over 50 198
    Tracking and Macros 199
    Fasting Over 50 203
    Keto Diet for Longevity 204
    Exercise for Women Over 50 in Support of Keto ... 206
    Tips and Tricks for Ketogenic Weight Loss 209

Chapter 3: Keto Food and Ketosis **214**
    Food Quality 214
    Foods to Eat 216
    Proteins 219
    Carbohydrates 223
    Nutritional Food List 228
    Spices and Sauces for Flavor 241

What Foods to Avoid 245

Keto Approved Sweeteners 248

Keto on a Budget 250

Keto Away From Home 252

Keto at Restaurants 254

Chapter 4: What are the Best Fats on Keto?..............**256**

Types of Fat...256

Omega-3, Omega-6, Omega-9 260

Fat Bombs 261

Chapter 5: Negative Moments in Keto **263**

Keto Flu...263

Constipation..265

Diarrhea 265

Insomnia 266

Diet Plateaus 267

Cholesterol and Keto 269

Chapter 6: Keto Recipes **272**

Breakfast 272

Keto-Friendly Breakfast Tortilla *272*

Breakfast Sandwich..*274*

Banana Nut Muffins *276*

Smoothies and Beverages 279

Coconut Green Smoothie *279*

Strawberry Smoothie..*280*

Keto Mojito *281*

Soup 283

- *Chicken and Riced Cauliflower Soup* *283*
- *Spicy Creamy Chicken Soup* *285*
- *Broccoli Cheese Soup* *287*

Sauces and Dips 289
- *Tzatziki* *289*
- *Satay Sauce* *290*
- *Thousand Island Salad Dressing* *291*
- *Hollandaise Sauce* *293*

Side Dishes 295
- *Mexican Cauliflower Rice* *295*
- *Green Beans and Bacon* *297*
- *Baked Spaghetti Squash* *298*

Snacks 300
- *Taco Flavored Cheddar Crisps* *300*
- *Keto Seed Crispy Crackers* *302*

Beef – Pork – Chicken 304
- *Slow Cooker Chilli* *304*
- *Chicken Parmesan* *306*
- *Baked Un-BBQ Ribs* *308*

Fish 310
- *Salmon skewers* *310*
- *Coconut Salmon with Napa Cabbage* *312*
- *Keto Tuna Casserole* *314*

Vegetarian 316
- *Cinnamon Crunch Cereal* *316*
- *Broccoli Cheese Fritters* *318*

Asian Noodle Salad *320*
　Dessert *322*
　　Cocoa Brownies *322*
　　Chocolate Chip Cookies *325*
　　Keto Brown Butter Pralines *327*
Conclusion **329**

Keto Vegan Cookbook for Beginners

The Ultimate Guide to Ketogenic & Plant-Based Diet with Easy and Healthy Low Carb Recipes for Rapid Weight Loss, Boost Energy & Reset your Body

Introduction

Congratulations on purchasing your copy of the *Keto-Vegan Cookbook for Beginners*. I'm thrilled to help guide you in this adventure in improving your health. You are well on your way to discovering many great recipes to delight your taste buds.

You will find recipes for all types of tastes within these pages; each recipe will provide you with estimated cooking time, serving size, and nutritional values. I have worked very hard to take a lot of the guesswork out so that you can simply cook and enjoy.

I wrote this cookbook because there was a gap that needed to be filled: there are many vegan and keto options, but either of them did not make me feel that I'm eating according to my goals. I spent so much time making substitutions to recipes, researching what to use in place of certain ingredients, and re-figuring the nutritional facts that it just made sense to develop an easy guide for all our Keto-Vegan friends.

If you are tired of starting a recipe only to find that you need to make adjustments or change ingredients, then this is the book for you. I have worked tirelessly to ensure every recipe meets my high standards of being a Keto-Vegan.

There are plenty of cookbooks on the Keto or Vegan diet, so

thanks again for choosing this one! Every effort was made to ensure that it is full of as much useful information as possible.

Chapter 1: Veganism

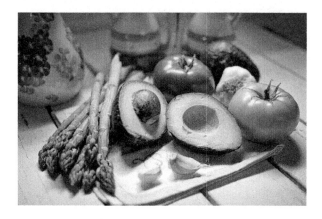

Veganism began in 1944 when a little group of vegetarians broke away to create the Vegan society. It was their choice not to consume any product that came from any animal. Some choose a vegan lifestyle for ethical reasons, such as the belief that all animal life is valuable, and they work to limit the exploitation of animals as much as possible. Some vegans choose this lifestyle for health reasons and others for environmental reasons.

When eating a vegan diet, these are some foods to avoid:

- Honey
- Fish
- Dairy
- Chicken
- Shellfish
- Meat

On the flip side of that, vegans still enjoy many of the

normal fan favorites, such as bean burritos, veggie burgers, pizza, smoothies, and chips just with a twist. Vegans typically swap out those meat-based options with things like the following:

- Seeds
- Nuts
- Tempeh
- Seitan
- Tofu
- Lentils
- Beans

Milk products are also replaced with plant-based milk and honey with plant sweeteners.

If you are living a vegan lifestyle, it is important to ensure that your body is still getting all the vitamins and minerals it needs. There are seven basic supplements I suggest you include when choosing this lifestyle. Always consult your nutritionist or doctor if you have questions.

- Vitamin B12 – Yes, you can get b12 from some plant-based options; however, scientists believe that vegans are at a higher risk of b12 deficiency. Too little b12 can lead to anemia. The daily recommended dosage is 2.4 mcg for adults.

- Vitamin D – this is the vitamin that helps you to absorb calcium and phosphorus in the gut. Vitamin D also has influence over many other processes, such as muscle recovery, memory, mood, and immune function. Consider taking a vitamin D2 or D3 supplement daily.

- Long-Chain Omega-3s – These are your fatty acids; they are important to the structural role for your eyes and brain. The recommended dose is to take a supplement containing EPA and DHA of 200 to 300 mg.

- Iodine – This is crucial for the function of your metabolism and the health of your thyroid. The recommended dosage for an adult is 150 mcg of iodine.

- Iron – This is essential for helping the body create new red blood cells and DNA, as well as carry oxygen into the blood. Low levels of iron can also result in fatigue. The recommended dosage is 8 milligrams for a male per day and 18 milligrams for a woman per day.

- Calcium – This mineral is essential for healthy teeth and bones, as well as the health of the heart. The recommended dosage amount is 1,000 mg per day.

- Zinc – This mineral is responsible for the repair of body cells, immune function, and metabolism. Insufficient zinc levels can result in diarrhea, hair loss, and developmental problems. The recommended dosage for zinc is 8 mg per day.

With all this being said, you can achieve many of these vitamins and nutrients through your plant-based diet. However, it is important to consider the use of supplements to offset the gaps between diet and body needs. Always remember to consult your health care professional.

Chapter 2: Ketogenic Diet

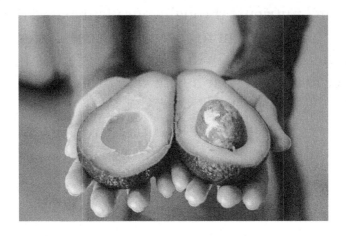

Keto is short for Ketogenic. A "Ketogenic Diet" is basically a low-carb diet. Through this diet, you are focusing your calorie intake on protein while reducing your calorie intake from fat and carbohydrates. There are specific food types that the body can digest easier than others. These would include things like sugar, soda, sweets, and white bread. Your body actually uses these sugary sources as fuel. Think of it like using regular gas in your car. It works great; however, when you put premium fuel, you often get a better mile per gallon ratio. The human body works the same way; the better fuel you give it, the more efficient it works. When starting out with keto, it can take three to four days before the body has "burned" off the sugary fuel. To get to that point, you will want to focus on eating 50 grams of carbs or less per day. Once that sugar fuel is gone, the body will then begin to break down protein and fat for energy. Some begin to see weight loss right away. This process is called ketosis, which is the body's natural way of creating fuel through ketones when there are not enough carbs to burn for energy.

The keto lifestyle is typically a short-term diet with focus on weight loss. Those living on a keto lifestyle have seen significant increase in weight loss compared to the other diets during the initial months. However, weight loss is not the only reason people are living on a keto lifestyle. There have been some research studies conducted claiming that keto may help people with other medical conditions, such as diabetes, heart disease, and even acne. Be sure to consult a doctor if you have any serious medical condition before starting the keto diet.

Those on the keto diet must avoid these types of food:

- Grains rice
- Low-fat dairy
- Sugars
- Starchy vegetables like potatoes, corn
- Trans fats
- Alcohol

On the other side, keto dieters enjoy:

- Vegetables like tomatoes, eggplants, asparagus, leafy greens, cucumber, Bell pepper
- Chicken, turkey venison, beef, seafood, eggs, natural cheese, whole milk ricotta cheese
- Oils, flaxseed, chia seed, pumpkin seed, sesame seed, nuts, and no-sugar kinds of butter.

Like the vegan diet, the ketogenic diet may be lacking on some minerals and vitamins, so taking supplements may be the best approach. Some of these are also listed under the vegan diet. Here are at least five supplements recommended when on a keto diet:

- Magnesium – This helps with your cellular functions, regulates the immune system, and strengthens the muscles and nerves. The recommended dosage is 310 mg.

- Calcium – The recommended dosage is also 1,000 mg per day.

- Iron – Take 8 milligrams a fay if you are a male and 18 milligrams if you are a woman.

- Vitamin D – Take vitamin D2 or D3, one tablet a day.

- Fiber – Fiber helps to keep your gut healthy and the GI tract running smooth. It is recommended to discuss with your health care professional for the appropriate dosage based on your body's needs.

You can get many of the vitamins and nutrients that your body needs from the keto diet. However, as we have mentioned earlier, it would still be better to fill the gaps that this lifestyle may create.

Chapter 3: Keto-Vegan Diet

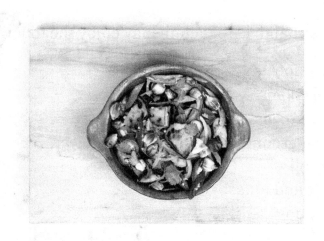

The keto-vegan lifestyle is one of the most restrictive lifestyles that suggest a very specific diet. However, it is possible to follow. In this lifestyle, you are focusing on a diet that is free of food products derived from animals. The diet is also low in carbohydrates. One of the key factors to success in this lifestyle is to eat not more than 5% of calories from carbohydrates. That would be approximately 50 grams of carbs in one day. However, many recommend staying at the lower end of 35 grams per day. Additionally, it is important to receive 70% of daily calories from plant-based fats and 25% from plant-based proteins.

Those on the keto-vegan diet should avoid these types of food:

- Grains, wheat, corn, rice
- Sugars – honey

- Fruit – apples, bananas
- Starches – potato, yams

On the other hand, keto dieters may enjoy the following:

- Vegan meats
- Mushrooms
- Leafy greens – kale, spinach
- Above-ground vegetables – cauliflower, zucchini, broccoli
- Seeds and nuts
- Avocados
- Berries
- Sea vegetables
- Sweeteners – stevia, monk fruit

Many studies have shown that a keto-vegan lifestyle provides health benefits. These benefits include lowering the risk of heart disease, greater mental health, improved vision, better stomach and gut health, and improved sleep. As always, make sure you are working with your healthcare professional to ensure you are getting all the vitamins and minerals that your body needs.

One thing is for sure; it is easier than before to live on a keto-vegan lifestyle with all the healthy food choices out there. There is also an abundance of alternatives for dairy and eggs that can help keep you on track with the keto portion of your life. The following chapters present the different recipes you can try while on the vegan-keto diet.

Chapter 4: Breakfast Choices

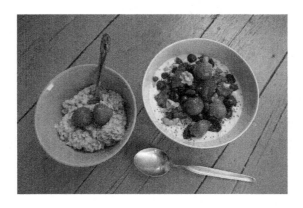

You can make a wide-range of breakfast treats, from tasty muffins to smoothies, to get your day kick-started in the right way.

Strawberry Porridge

Total Prep & Cooking Time: 9 min.
Yields: 2 Servings
Nutrition Facts: Calories: 374 | Proteins: 11 g | Carbohydrates: 9 g | Fats: 33 g

Ingredients

1/3 c. coconut milk, full-fat canned
½ c. water
1 tbsp. coconut flour
¼ c. hemp seeds
½ c. flacked unsweetened coconut
2 strawberries sliced

½ tbs. ground cinnamon
1 t. vanilla
1-2 teaspoons sweetener of your choice.

Follow these simple steps:

1. Add milk, water, coconut, coconut flour, & hemp seed to a pan for cooking on the stove.
2. In this pan, allow these ingredients to a come to a boil for approximately 2 minutes, simmering until thick.
3. Add cinnamon & vanilla and combine until well-mixed and put in a heat-resistant bowl.
4. Slice the strawberries and place on top of the porridge and sprinkle the sweetener of your choice across the top.
5. Enjoy with additional milk as needed.

Gingerbread Porridge

Total Prep & Cooking Time: 9 min.
Yields: 2 Servings
Nutrition Facts: Calories: 374 | Proteins: 11 g | Carbohydrates: 9 g | Fats: 33 g

Ingredients

1/3 c. coconut milk, full-fat, canned
½ c. water
1 tbsp. coconut flour
¼ c. hemp seeds
½ c. flacked unsweetened coconut
1 ½ t. ground ginger
1 t. of the following:
- ground cloves
- ground nutmeg
- vanilla

½ tbsp. ground cinnamon
1-2 teaspoons sweetener of your choice

Optional Toppings
Almond butter, chopped walnuts/pecans, cranberries

Follow these simple steps:

1. In a medium saucepan, add the milk, water, coconut, coconut flour, & hemp seed.
2. Bring these ingredients to a boil, allowing to simmer 2 minutes or until thickened.

3. Add cinnamon, vanilla ginger, cloves, nutmeg, and combine until well-mixed and put in a heat-resistant bowl.
4. Sprinkle sweetener and any optional toppings of your choice across the top.
5. Mix and enjoy with additional milk as needed.

Overnight Strawberry Cheesecake Porridge

Total Prep & Cooking Time: 10 min.
Yields: 1 Servings
Nutrition Facts: Calories: 275 | Proteins: 8 g | Carbohydrates: 16 g | Fats: 17 g

Ingredients

¼ c. fresh strawberries
½ c. coconut milk
2 tbsp. of the following:
- coconut yogurt
- ground flaxseed
- chia seeds
- sweetener of your choice

1 tbsp. of the following:
- almond flour
- shredded unsweetened coconut

Follow these simple steps:

1. Mix almond flour, unsweetened coconut, sweetener, chia seed, and flaxseed in a shallow bowl.

2. Next, pour ¼ cup of the coconut milk with dry contents and combine well.
3. Refrigerate overnight.
4. Before serving, add the remaining milk until the mixture becomes thick and creamy.
5. Layer the yogurt and strawberries on top.
6. Mix and enjoy.

Blueberry Quinoa Porridge

Total Prep & Cooking Time: 20 min.
Yields: 2 Servings
Nutrition Facts: Calories: 374 | Proteins: 11 g | Carbohydrates: 9 g | Fats: 33 g

Ingredients

1 c. blueberries
1/8 t. cinnamon
¼ t. vanilla
1 tbsp. sweetener of your choice
2 c. almond milk
1 c. uncooked quinoa

Optional Toppings
Chia seeds, hemp seeds, hazelnuts

Follow these simple steps:

1. In a saucepan, add milk and quinoa.

2. Heat milk and quinoa at low heat for roughly 10 minutes, stirring to prevent scorching.
3. Slowly combine vanilla, cinnamon, and sugar and cook for 5 minutes or when the quinoa soft.
4. Take away from the heat and place in serving bowls.
5. Top with blueberries and sprinkle sweetener of your choice across the top.
6. Mix and enjoy.

Blueberry Chia Pudding

Total Prep & Cooking Time: 8 hours 10 min.
Yields: 3 Servings
Nutrition Facts: Calories: 374 | Proteins: 11 g | Carbohydrates: 9 g | Fats: 33 g

Ingredients

1/8 t. cinnamon
½ t. vanilla
2 c. almond milk, unsweetened
1 tbsp. maple syrup
1/3 c. blueberries
6 tbsp. chia seeds, fresh

Follow these simple steps:

1. Combine the chia seeds, blueberries, syrup, milk, vanilla, and cinnamon into a blender, blending into a silky consistency.
2. Separate mixture into 3 glasses or ramekins.

3. Chill overnight or until set, approximately 8 hours.
4. Enjoy it chilled.

Pro Tip:
Using frozen blueberries will allow the mixture to have a little more texture

Almond Flour Muffins

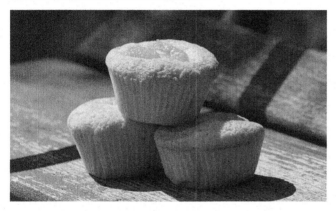

Total Prep & Cooking Time: 10 min.
Yields: 4 regular size Muffins or 14 Mini Muffins Servings
Nutrition Facts: Calories: 217 | Proteins: 11 g | Carbohydrates: 9 g | Fats: 33 g

Ingredients

¼ t. salt
½ tbsp. baking powder
1 flax egg
¼ c. almond milk
1 tbsp. stevia (or your sweetener of choice)
1 c. almond flour

Olive oil for greasing muffin pan.

Optional add-in
Crushed, walnuts, blueberries, sugar-free chocolate chips

Follow these simple steps:

1. Set the oven to preheat at 350.
2. Grease the muffin pan with olive oil.
3. Combine baking powder, stevia, salt, and almond flour in a mixing bowl. Mix completely.
4. Slowly add the flax egg and almond milk and mix well
5. If adding any add-ins, add them at this point (crushed walnuts, blueberries, chocolate chips).
6. Using a ¼ c. measuring cup, fill each muffin tin approximately 2/3 full.
7. Carefully slide into the oven and cook for 10 minutes (mini size) or 15 minutes (regular size).
8. Take it from oven and place in a cool area to allow muffins to cool while still in the tin for about 10 minutes. Then, carefully remove the muffins using a knife to loosen them from the sides of the tin.

Bulletproof Tea

Total Prep & Cooking Time: 2 min.
Yields: 1 Serving
Nutrition Facts: Calories: 151 | Proteins: 0 g | Carbohydrates: 1 g | Fats: 17 g

Ingredients

1/8 t. ground cinnamon
1 tbsp. of the following:
- coconut milk
- coconut oil

1-2 t. black tea
8 oz. boiling water
Sweetener of your choice

Follow these simple steps:

1. Begin by boiling 8 oz of water.
2. Then add the black tea to steep according to your package directions.
3. Once the tea is done steeping, pour it into a blender then add coconut oil, coconut milk, cinnamon, and a sweetener of your choice.
4. Blend approximately 30 seconds or until smooth.
5. Pour into a cup and enjoy.

Bulletproof Coffee

Total Prep & Cooking Time: 3 min.
Yields: 2 Serving
Nutrition Facts: Calories: 354 | Proteins: 4.4 g | Carbohydrates: 4.7 g | Fats: 37.2 g

Ingredients

2 c. strong coffee
¼ cup almond milk, unsweetened
2 tbsp. coconut oil, extra virgin
1 oz. raw cacao butter
1 1/2 tbsp. almond butter

Follow these simple steps:

1. In a microwave-safe pitcher, heat cacao butter, coconut oil, and almond butter until melted; this may take approximately 20 seconds.
2. Add the almond milk slowly and stir.
3. Microwave an additional 30 seconds.
4. Remove from the microwave and add coffee. Blend with a handheld froth machine or blender until creamy.
5. Pour into a cup and enjoy.

Coconut Pancakes

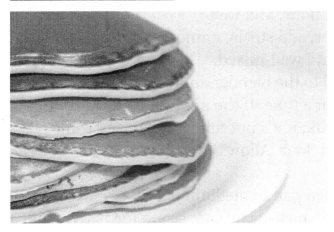

Total Prep & Cooking Time: 10 min.
Yields: 4 Serving
Nutrition Facts: Calories: 491 | Proteins: 11 g | Carbohydrates: 41.9 g | Fats: 33 g

Ingredients

1 t. cinnamon
1 ½ c. coconut milk
1/3 c. coconut flour
1 big banana
1 c. quinoa flakes
1 serving liquid stevia
1 t. baking powder
2/3 c. almond flour

Follow these simple steps:

1. Combine in a big glass bowl the baking powder with both types of flour. Mix well.
2. In the blender, add stevia, quinoa flakes, banana, and cinnamon until well-mixed.
3. Add big bowl to the blender and begin adding coconut milk ½ cup at a time. If the mixture is thick, add additional milk; if it's not thin enough, add some more almond flour. Allow the batter to rest for about 5 minutes.
4. Warm a big flat pan to medium heat.
5. Using a ¼ cup measuring cup, scoop the batter from the blender. Pour in the skillet, covering to cook for 2 minutes or when bubbles begin to form. Flip and repeat.
6. Enjoy warm.

Flaxseed Pancakes

Total Prep & Cooking Time: 10 min.
Yields: 4 Serving
Nutrition Facts: Calories: 239 | Proteins: 12.6 g | Carbohydrates: 8.7 g | Fats: 18.9 g

Ingredients

¼ t of the following:
- vanilla
- baking soda

1 t. apple cider vinegar
1 flax egg
¼ c. ground golden flaxseed meal
1 tbsp. almond milk
Dash of cinnamon & nutmeg
Pinch of sea salt

Follow these simple steps:

1. Incorporate all of the above in a big glass bowl and mix. The batter should be a thicker mixture and sticky. If it doesn't spread well in the pan, add more milk.
2. Warm a flat pan or griddle to medium heat. Using olive oil, grease the pan to prevent the pancakes from sticking.
3. Using a spoon, scoop the batter from the bowl and form 2-3 pancakes in your pan. Use the spoon to help flatten out the batter.

4. Cook 2 minutes or until bubbles are forming. Flip and repeat; be sure to keep a close eye on these, so they do not burn.
5. Enjoy warm.

Berry and Nut Cereal

Total Prep & Cooking Time: 15 min.
Yields: 2 Serving
Nutrition Facts: Calories: 776 | Proteins: 10.8 g | Carbohydrates: 27.7 g | Fats: 73.3 g

Ingredients

1/3 c. of the following:
- strawberries
- blueberries
- toasted flaxseed
- crushed walnut pieces

2 c. almond milk
½ c. shredded unsweetened coconut
Pinch of salt

Follow these simple steps:

1. In a saucepan, toast nuts and salt over low to medium heat; cook for approximately 2 minutes.
2. Add shredded coconut and stir constantly to prevent burning; do this for about 1 minute.
3. Once toasted, add almond milk and stir to combine.
4. Pull from the heat and divide into 2 bowls.

5. Divide the strawberries and blueberries between bowls
6. Sprinkle with a sweetener of your choice.
7. Enjoy warm.

Peanut Butter Fudgy Brownies

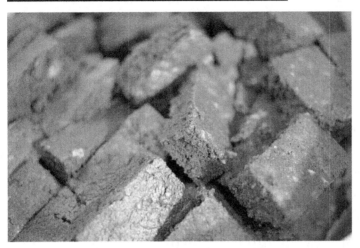

Total Prep & Cooking Time: 20 min.
Yields: 9 Serving
Nutrition Facts: Calories: 321 | Proteins: 9.6 g | Carbohydrates: 30.1 g | Fats: 22.5 g

Ingredients

2/3 c. chocolate chips
¾ c. of the following:
- brown sugar
- peanut butter
- almond milk

½ t. of each:
- salt
- baking powder

¼ c. cacao powder
1 t. vanilla
1 c. almond flour
2 tbsp. ground flax
5 tbsp. water

Follow these simple steps:

1. Begin by bringing the oven temperature to 350.
2. While the oven is preheating, combine in a bowl the ground flax and water, allowing these to sit for approximately 5 minutes to thicken.
3. Next, in a big mixing bowl, add salt, baking powder, cacao powder, and almond flour.
4. In the center of the mixture, form a well and add in the thickened flax water mixture, vanilla, coconut sugar, peanut butter, and milk.
5. Stir until the mixture forms a nice thick batter.
6. Next, fold in the chocolate chips.
7. In a 9x9 greased baking dish, pour the batter using a spatula to even it out.
8. On top, add 5 dollops of peanut butter, then using a knife, swirl the peanut butter into the brownie batter.
9. Place brownies in the preheated oven, baking for 20 minutes. Allow the brownies to reduce in temperature in the pan for 10 minutes.
10. After this, you can place the yummy treats on a cooling rack. Slice and enjoy!

Vanilla Golden Turmeric Cereal

Total Prep & Cooking Time: 55 min.
Yields: 2 Serving
Nutrition Facts: Calories: 585 | Proteins: 9.4 g | Carbohydrates: 84.5 g | Fats: 21.6 g

Ingredients

1 c. almond milk unsweetened vanilla silk
3 tbsp. coconut oil melted
¼ t. ground cloves
½ t. ginger
1 tbsp. of the following:
- turmeric
- cinnamon
- vanilla

6 tbsp. maple syrup
1 t. Himalayan salt
3 tbsp. ground flaxseed
3 c. quinoa flakes

Follow these simple steps:

1. Begin by bringing the oven temperature to 350.
2. Combine the cloves, ginger, turmeric, cinnamon, vanilla, syrup, salt flax, and quinoa flakes in a big mixing bowl.
3. Move to a cookie sheet in an even layer, approximately ½ inch thick. Place the mixture in the oven, baking for 40 minutes. Every 10 minutes, stir to get even cooking and prevent the edges from burning.

4. Let it cool completely.
5. Add them to the bowls and pour almond milk over the top.
6. Enjoy.

Fudge Oatmeal

Total Prep & Cooking Time: 5 min.
Yields: 1 Serving
Nutrition Facts: Calories: 262 | Proteins: 9 g | Carbohydrates: 14 g | Fats: 18 g

Ingredients

½ t. vanilla
2 tbsp. chocolate chips
2 t. cocoa powder
2 tbsp. of the following:
- ground flaxseed
- chia seed
- unsweetened shredded coconut
- sweetener of your choice

½ c. hot water
¾ c. coconut milk

Follow these simple steps:

1. Add ground flaxseed, chia seed, shredded coconut, and sweetener of your choice to a bowl and mix well.
2. Pour ½ cup of hot water into the dry ingredients and mix well. It will be thick.

3. Add ½ cup coconut milk to make a creamy oatmeal base.
4. Next, add ¼ cup milk, vanilla, chocolate chips, and cocoa powder.
5. Heat over the stovetop or in the microwave until the chocolate chips have melted.
6. Top with the reaming chocolate chips and enjoy.
7. Enjoy.

Raspberry Almond Smoothie

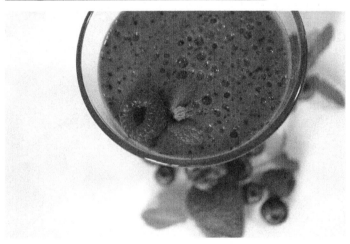

Total Prep & Cooking Time: 5 min.
Yields: 1 Serving
Nutrition Facts: Calories: 156 | Proteins: 2.8 g | Carbohydrates: 26.6 g | Fats: 5.4 g

Ingredients

3 t. maple syrup
½ c. raspberry

2 c. almond milk unsweetened vanilla silk

Follow these simple steps:

1. Combine in a blender the almond milk, raspberries, and syrup and blend for 3 minutes or until smooth. If it seems too dense, i.e., it's difficult to drink, add an additional ¼ cup of milk.
2. Enjoy.

Vanilla Overnight Oats

Total Prep & Cooking Time: 5 min.
Yields: 1 Serving
Nutrition Facts: Calories: 132 | Proteins: 6.5 g | Carbohydrates: 4.9 g | Fats: 1 g

Ingredients

½ t. vanilla
3 to 4 drops liquid stevia
1 tbsp. chia seed
½ c. hemp hearts
2/3 c. almond milk unsweetened vanilla silk

Follow these simple steps:

1. Add hemp hearts, chia seed, stevia, vanilla, and ½ the milk to a bowl; mix it until well-combined.
2. Cover and refrigerate overnight or for a minimum of 8 hours.

3. Remove from the fridge, divide into 2 bowls, and enjoy with a splash of milk.

Cinnamon Overnight Oats

Total Prep & Cooking Time: 5 min.
Yields: 1 Serving
Nutrition Facts: Calories: 132 | Proteins: 6.5 g | Carbohydrates: 4.9 g | Fats: 1 g

Ingredients

½ t. vanilla
½ tbsp. cinnamon
3 to 4 drops liquid stevia
1 tbsp. chia seed
½ c. hemp hearts
2/3 c. almond milk unsweetened vanilla silk

Follow these simple steps:

1. Add hemp hearts, chia seed, stevia, cinnamon, vanilla, and ½ the milk to a bowl; mix the ingredients until well-combined.
2. Cover and refrigerate overnight or for 8 hours.
3. When ready for serving, take it out of the fridge, scoop some into a bowl, and enjoy with the remaining milk.

Pumpkin Spice Overnight Oats

Total Prep & Cooking Time: 5 min.
Yields: 1 Serving
Nutrition Facts: Calories: 132 | Proteins: 6.5 g | Carbohydrates: 4.9 g | Fats: 1 g

Ingredients

½ t. vanilla
¾ t. pumpkin spice
3 to 4 drops liquid stevia
1 tbsp. chia seed
2 tbsp. canned pumpkin puree
½ c. hemp hearts
1/3 c. of the following:
- brewed coffee
- almond milk unsweetened vanilla silk

Follow these simple steps:

1. In a bowl with a lid, add all the ingredients, mixing until well-combined.
2. Cover and refrigerate overnight or 8 hours.
3. Remove from the fridge and add additional milk until the oats reach your desired consistency.
4. Divide into 2 bowls and enjoy.

Smoothie Bowl

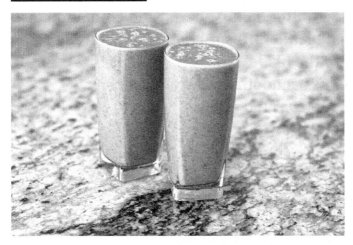

Total Prep & Cooking Time: 15 min.
Yields: 2 Serving
Nutrition Facts: Calories: 253 | Proteins: 6.5 g | Carbohydrates: 4.9 g | Fats: 1 g

Ingredients

1 t. ground cinnamon
3 tbsp. hemp hearts
2 tbsp. almond butter
1 c. of the following:
- vanilla unsweetened almond milk
- frozen blueberries
- frozen spinach

½ c. of the following:
- frozen zucchini
- frozen cauliflower

Follow these simple steps:

1. Throw the cauliflower, zucchini, spinach, blueberries, milk, almond butter, hemp hearts, and cinnamon into a high-speed blender. Ensure the frozen ingredients are closest to the blades.
2. Blend until it's a smooth, creamy consistency.
3. Divide into 2 bowls and enjoy.

Eggy Surprise Scramble

Total Prep & Cooking Time: 10 min.
Yields: 2 Serving
Nutrition Facts: Calories: 206 | Proteins: 20.3 g | Carbohydrates: 4 g | Fats: 13.1 g

Ingredients

1/3 c. soy milk
¼ t. of the following:
- onion powder
- black salt (Kala Namak)

½ t. of the following:
- garlic powder
- paprika
- turmeric

1 t. Dijon mustard
1 tbsp. vegan butter
2 tbsp. nutritional yeast
8oz extra firm tofu

Optional ingredients

- black pepper
- chives
- fried Tomatoes
- sliced Avocado

Follow these simple steps:

1. With a fork, chop the tofu into nice big chunks.
2. Combine in the mixing bowl garlic powder, onion powder, black pepper, salt, mustard, paprika, yeast, and turmeric. Once mixed well, whisk in the soy milk to create a sauce.
3. Warm over a medium heat a skillet, adding butter and stirring to melt.
4. Next, apply the tofu and fry until a light golden color; be careful not to over-scramble the tofu.
5. Add the sauce mixture to the tofu and fry until the sauce has been mostly absorbed by the tofu.
6. Remove it from skillet and transfer to a plate; top it with optional ingredients and enjoy.

Bagels

Total Prep & Cooking Time: 50 min.
Yields: 6 Serving
Nutrition Facts: Calories: 209 | Proteins: 6.6 g | Carbohydrates: 2 g | Fats: 16.4 g

Ingredients

Pinch of salt
1 t. baking powder
¼ c. psyllium husks
½ c of the following:
- tahini
- ground flaxseed

1 c. water
Optional ingredients
Almond butter, fresh fruit

Follow these simple steps:

1. Set the oven to 375 heat setting.
2. In a mixing bowl medium in size, add salt, flaxseed, baking powder, and psyllium husk.
3. Whisk until well-combined.
4. In a little bowl, add water and tahini and whisk until combined.
5. Add the wet ingredients in the small bowl to the medium bowl and knead until the dough is well-worked and has a uniform consistency.
6. Using your hands, divide the dough into six equal parts.

7. Hand-form each bagel into a 4-inch diameter approximately ¼-inch thick. Place on a cooki and cut the center out (optional), or use a donut pan to form your bagels.
8. Bake them until golden brown or approximately 40 minutes.
9. Take out of the oven and allow to cool slightly or enjoy warm.

Cinnamon Roll Muffins

Total Prep & Cooking Time: 20 min.
Yields: 12 Serving
Nutrition Facts: Calories: 112 | Proteins: 5 g | Carbohydrates: 3g | Fats: 9 g

Ingredients

½ c. of the following:
- coconut oil
- pumpkin puree
- almond butter
- almond flour

1 tbsp. cinnamon
1 t. baking powder
2 scoops vanilla protein powder

For the Icing:

2 t. lemon juice
1 tbsp. sweetener of choice
1/4 c. of the following:

- coconut butter
- milk of choice

Follow these simple steps:

1. Set the oven to 350 setting.
2. Prepare your 12-count muffin pan with muffin liners.
3. Combine protein powder, cinnamon, flour, and baking powder, combining well in a big mixing bowl.
4. Next, add the coconut oil, pumpkin, and butter and mix until fully incorporated.
5. Divide the batter into muffin liners.
6. Slide into the oven, baking for 10 to 15 minutes.
7. After removing from the oven, leave the muffins in tin to cool for five minutes then carefully place on a cooling rack. While cooling, prepare the icing by mixing lemon juice, sweetener, coconut butter, and milk.
8. Drizzle over cooled muffin tops; allow them to sit for 2 to 5 minutes while icing the firms.
9. Serve and enjoy.

Chapter 5: Lunch & Dinner Favorites

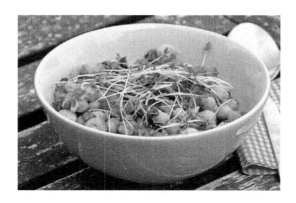

It's time to kick up your taste buds with these dishes for lunch or dinner

Mushroom Steak

Total Prep & Cooking Time: 1 hr. 30 min.
Yields: 8 Servings
Nutrition Facts: Calories: 87 | Carbohydrates: 6.2 g | Proteins: 3 g | Fats: 6.2 g

Ingredients:

1 tbsp. of the following:
- fresh lemon juice
- olive oil, extra virgin

2 tbsp. coconut oil
3 thyme sprigs
8 medium Portobello mushrooms

For Sauce:

1 ½ t. of the following:
- minced garlic
- minced peeled fresh ginger

2 tbsp. of the following:
- light brown sugar
- mirin

½ c. low-sodium soy sauce

Follow these simple steps:

1. For the sauce, combine all the sauce ingredients, along with ¼ cup water into a little pan and simmer to cook. Cook using a medium heat until it reduces to a glaze, approximately 15 to 20 minutes, then remove from the heat.
2. For the mushrooms, bring the oven to 350 heat setting.
3. Using a skillet, melt coconut oil and olive oil, cooking the mushrooms on each side for about 3 minutes.
4. Next, arrange the mushrooms in a single layer on a sheet for baking and season with lemon juice, salt, and pepper.
5. Carefully slide into the oven and roast for 5 minutes. Let it rest for 2 minutes.
6. Plate and drizzle the sauce over the mushrooms.
7. Enjoy.

Spicy Grilled Tofu Steak

Total Prep & Cooking Time: 20 min.
Yields: 4 Servings
Nutrition Facts: Calories: 155 | Carbohydrates: 7.6 g | Proteins: 9.9 g | Fats: 11.8 g

Ingredients:
1 tbsp. of the following:
- chopped scallion
- chopped cilantro
- soy sauce
- hoisin sauce

2 tbsp. oil
¼ t. of the following:
- salt
- garlic powder
- red chili pepper powder
- ground Sichuan peppercorn powder

½ t. cumin
1 pound firm tofu

Follow these simple steps:

1. Place the tofu on a plate and drain the excess liquid for about 10 minutes.
2. Slice drained tofu into ¾ thick stakes.
3. Stir the cumin, Sichuan peppercorn, chili powder, garlic powder, and salt in a mixing bowl until well-incorporated.
4. In another little bowl, combine soy sauce, hoisin, and

1 teaspoon of oil.
5. Heat a skillet to medium temperature with oil, then carefully place the tofu in the skillet.
6. Sprinkle the spices over the tofu, distributing equally across all steaks. Cook for 3-5 minutes, flip, and put spice on the other side. Cook for an additional 3 minutes.
7. Brush with sauce and plate.
8. Sprinkle some scallion and cilantro and enjoy.

Piquillo Salsa Verde Steak

Total Prep & Cooking Time: 25 min.
Yields: 8 Servings
Nutrition Facts: Calories: 427 | Carbohydrates: 67.5 g | Proteins: 14.2 g | Fats: 14.6 g

Ingredients:
4 – ½ inch thick slices of ciabatta
18 oz. firm tofu, drained
5 tbsp. olive oil, extra virgin
Pinch of cayenne
½ t. cumin, ground
1 ½ tbsp. sherry vinegar
1 shallot, diced
8 piquillo peppers (can be from a jar) – drained and cut to ½ inch strips
3 tbsp. of the following:
- parsley, finely chopped
- capers, drained and chopped

Follow these simple steps:

1. Place the tofu on a plate to drain the excess liquid, and then slice into 8 rectangle pieces.
2. You can either prepare your grill or use a grill pan. If using a grill pan, preheat the grill pan.
3. Mix 3 tablespoons of olive oil, cayenne, cumin, vinegar, shallot, parsley, capers, and piquillo peppers in a medium bowl to make our salsa verde. Season to preference with salt and pepper.
4. Using a paper towel, dry the tofu slices.
5. Brush olive oil on each side, seasoning with salt and pepper lightly.
6. Place the bread on the grill and toast for about 2 minutes using medium-high heat.
7. Next, grill the tofu, cooking each side for about 3 minutes or until the tofu is heated through.
8. Place the toasted bread on the plate then the tofu on top of the bread.
9. Gently spoon out the salsa verde over the tofu and serve.

Butternut Squash Steak

Total Prep & Cooking Time: 50 min.
Yields: 4 Servings
Nutrition Facts: Calories: 300 | Carbohydrates: 46 g | Proteins: 5.3 g | Fats: 10.6 g

Ingredients:
2 tbsp. coconut yogurt
½ t. sweet paprika
1 ¼ c. low-sodium vegetable broth
1 sprig thyme
1 finely chopped garlic clove
1 big thinly sliced shallot
1 tbsp. margarine
2 tbsp. olive oil, extra virgin
Salt and pepper to liking

Follow these simple steps:

1. Bring the oven to 375 heat setting.
2. Cut the squash, lengthwise, into 4 steaks.
3. Carefully core one side of each squash with a paring knife in a crosshatch pattern.
4. Using a brush, coat with olive oil each side of the steak then season generously with salt and pepper.
5. In an oven-safe, non-stick skillet, bring 2 tablespoons of olive oil to a warm temperature.
6. Place the steaks on the skillet with the cored side down and cook at medium temperature until browned, approximately 5 minutes.

7. Flip and repeat on the other side for about 3 minutes.
8. Place the skillet into the oven to roast the squash for 7 minutes.
9. Take out from the oven, placing on a plate and covering with aluminum foil to keep warm.
10. Using the previously used skillet, add thyme, garlic, and shallot, cooking at medium heat. Stir frequently for about 2 minutes.
11. Add brandy and cook for an additional minute.
12. Next, add paprika and whisk the mixture together for 3 minutes.
13. Add in the yogurt seasoning with salt and pepper.
14. Plate the steaks and spoon the sauce over the top.
15. Garnish with parsley and enjoy!

Cauliflower Steak Kicking Corn

Total Prep & Cooking Time: 60 min.
Yields: 6 Servings
Nutrition Facts: Calories: 153 | Carbohydrates: 15 g | Proteins: 4 g | Fats: 10 g

Ingredients:
2 t. capers, drained
4 scallions, chopped
1 red chili, minced
¼ c. vegetable oil
2 ears of corn, shucked
2 big cauliflower heads
Salt and pepper to taste

Follow these simple steps:

1. Heat the oven to 375 degrees.
2. Boil a pot of water, about 4 cups, using the maximum heat setting available.
3. Add corn in the saucepan, cooking approximately 3 minutes or until tender.
4. Drain and allow the corn to cool, then slice the kernels away from the cob.
5. Warm 2 tablespoons of vegetable oil in a skillet.
6. Combine the chili pepper with the oil, cooking for approximately 30 seconds.
7. Next, combine the scallions, sautéing with the chili pepper until soft.
8. Mix in the corn and capers in the skillet and cook for approximately 1 minute to blend the flavors. Then

remove from heat.
9. Warm 1 tablespoon of vegetable oil in a skillet. Once warm, begin to place cauliflower steaks to the pan, 2 to 3 at a time. Season to your liking with salt and cook over medium heat for 3 minutes or until lightly browned.
10. Once cooked, slide onto the cookie sheet and repeat step 5 with the remaining cauliflower.
11. Take the corn mixture and press into the spaces between the florets of the cauliflower.
12. Bake for 25 minutes.
13. Serve warm and enjoy!

Pistachio Watermelon Steak

Total Prep & Cooking Time: 10 min.
Yields: 4 Servings
Nutrition Facts: Calories: 67 | Carbohydrates: 3.8 g | Proteins: 1.6 g | Fats: 5.9 g

Ingredients:
Microgreens
Pistachios chopped
Malden sea salt
1 tbsp. olive oil, extra virgin
1 watermelon
Salt to taste

Follow these simple steps:

1. Begin by cutting the ends of the watermelon.
2. Carefully peel the skin from the watermelon along the white outer edge.
3. Slice the watermelon into 4 slices, approximately 2 inches thick.
4. Trim the slices, so they are rectangular in shape approximately 2 x4 inches.
5. Heat a skillet to medium heat add 1 tablespoon of olive oil.
6. Add watermelon steaks and cook until the edges begin to caramelize.
7. Plate and top with pistachios and microgreens.
8. Sprinkle with Malden salt.
9. Serve warm and enjoy!

BBQ Ribs

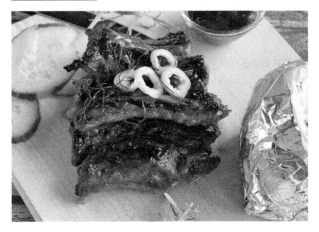

Total Prep & Cooking Time: 45 min.
Yields: 2 Servings
Nutrition Facts: Calories: 649 | Carbohydrates: 114 g | Proteins: 34.8 g | Fats: 11.1 g

Ingredients:
2 drops liquid smoke
2 tbsp. of the following:
- soy sauce
- tahini

1 c. of the following:
- water
- wheat gluten

1 tbsp. of the following:
- garlic powder
- onion powder
- lemon pepper

2 t. chipotle powder

For the Sauce:
2 chipotle peppers in adobo, minced
1 tbsp. of the following:
- vegan Worcestershire sauce
- lemon juice
- horseradish
- onion powder
- garlic powder
- ground pepper

1 t. dry mustard
2 tbsp. sweetener of your choice
5 tbsp. brown sugar
½ c. apple cider vinegar
2 c. ketchup
1 c. water
1 freshly squeezed orange juice

Follow these simple steps:

1. Set the oven to 350 heat setting, and prepare the grill charcoal as recommended for this, but gas will work as well.
2. Combine soy sauce, tahini, water, and liquid smoke in a bowl. Then set this mixture to the side in a mixing bowl.
3. Next, use a big glass bowl to mix chipotle powder, onion powder, lemon pepper, garlic powder; combine well then whisk in the ingredients from the little bowl.
4. Add the wheat gluten and mix until it comes to a gooey consistency.

5. Grease a standard-size loaf pan and transfer the mixture to the loaf pan. Smooth it out so that the rib mixture fits flat in the pan.
6. Bake for 30 minutes.
7. While the mixture is baking, make the BBQ sauce. To make the sauce, combine all the sauce ingredients in a pot. Allow the mixture to simmer its way to the boiling point to combine the flavors, and as soon as it boils, decrease the heat to the minimum setting. Let it be for 10 more minutes.
8. Cautiously take the rib out of the oven and slide onto a plate.
9. Coat the top rib mixture with the BBQ Sauce and place on the grill.
10. Coat the other side of the rib mixture with BBQ Sauce and grill for 6 minutes
11. Flip and grill the other side for an additional 6 minutes.
12. Serve warm and enjoy!

Spicy Veggie Steaks With veggies

Total Prep & Cooking Time: 45 mins.
Yields: 4 Servings
Nutrition Facts: Calories: 458 | Carbohydrates: 65.5 g | Proteins: 39.1 g | Fats: 7.6 g

Ingredients:
1 ¾ c. vital wheat gluten
½ c. vegetable stock
¼ t. liquid smoke
1 tbsp. Dijon mustard
1 t. paprika
½ c. tomato paste
2 tbsp. soy sauce
½ t. oregano
¼ t. of the following:
- coriander powder
- cumin

1 t. of the following:
- onion powder
- garlic powder

¼ c. nutritional yeast
¾ c. canned chickpeas

Marinade:
½ t. red pepper flakes
2 cloves garlic, minced
2 tbsp. soy sauce
1 tbsp. lemon juice, freshly squeezed
¼ c. maple syrup

For skewers:
15 skewers, soaked in water for 30 minutes if wooden
¾ t. salt
8 oz. zucchini or yellow summer squash
¼ t. ground black pepper
1 tbsp. olive oil
1 red onion, medium

Follow these simple steps:

1. In a food processor, add chickpeas, vegetable stock, liquid smoke, Dijon mustard, pepper, paprika, tomato paste, soy sauce, oregano, coriander, cumin, onion powder, garlic, and natural yeast. Process until the ingredients are well-mixed.
2. Add the vital wheat gluten to a big mixing bowl, and pour the contents from the food processor into the center. Mix with a spoon until a soft dough is formed.
3. Knead the dough for approximately 2 minutes; do not over knead.
4. Once the dough is firm and stretchy, flatten it to create 4 equal-sized steaks.
5. Individually wrap the steaks in tin foil; be sure not to wrap the steaks too tightly, as they will expand when steaming.
6. Steam for 20 minutes. To steam, you can use any steamer you like or a basket over boiling water.
7. While steaming, prepare the marinade. In a bowl, whisk the red pepper, garlic, soy sauce, lemon juice, and syrup. Reserve half of the sauce for brushing

during grilling.
8. Prepare the skewers. Cut the onion and zucchini or yellow squash into 1/2-inch chunks.
9. In a glass bowl, add the red onion, zucchini, and yellow squash then coat with olive oil, pepper, and salt to taste. Place the vegetables on the skewers.
10. After the steaks have steamed for 20 minutes, unwrap and place on a cookie sheet. Pour the marinade over the steaks, fully covering them.
11. Bring your skewers, steaks, and glaze to the grill. Place the skewers on the grill over direct heat. Brush skewers with glaze. Grill for approximately 3 minutes then flip.
12. Place the steaks directly on the grill, glaze side down, and brush the top with additional glaze. Cook to your desired doneness.
13. Serve warm and enjoy!

Tofu Seitan

Total Prep & Cooking Time: 1 hr, 40 mins.
Yields: 6 Servings
Nutrition Facts: Calories: 159 | Carbohydrates: 8 g | Proteins: 26 g | Fats: 2 g

Ingredients:
½ t. salt
1 t. garlic, powdered
2 t. vegetable broth
1 tbsp. onion, powdered
2 tbsp. of the following
- nutritional yeast
- water

1 ¼ c. tofu
1 ½ c. vital wheat gluten

Follow these simple steps:

1. Stir together the ingredients above in a bowl until a dough forms.
2. Lightly dust the countertop and your hands with wheat gluten. Using the counter service, form a ball out of the dough. Be careful not to knead it because it might make the seitan tough.
3. Once the ball is formed, cut it into 6 equal pieces.
4. Using your fingers press each ball into an oval shape, about 4x6 inches.
5. With a steamer basket placed inside a big pot, add water into the bottom of the pot and bring it to a

rolling boil.
6. Place the seitan into the steamer basket; if they overlap, brush them with oil to prevent them from sticking.
7. Cover and steam for approximately 12 minutes then flip so that both sides steam evenly.
8. Once steamed on both sides, remove and allow cooling for a minimum of 1 hour.
9. The tenders are fully cooked at this point, so you can re-heat them or toss them on the grill with your favorite sauce, or you can eat them cold over leafy greens.
10. Enjoy!

Stuffed Zucchini

Total Prep & Cooking Time: 30 mins.
Yields: 4 Servings
Nutrition Facts: Calories: 159 | Carbohydrates: 8 g | Proteins: 26 g | Fats: 2 g

Ingredients:
1 ½ c. black beans, drained
¼ t. chili powder
½ of the following:
- sea salt
- cumin, ground

1 of the following
- clove garlic, minced
- red bell pepper, diced
- red onion, diced

1 tbsp. olive oil, extra virgin
4 medium zucchini

For the Sauce
¼ t. of the following:
- chili powder
- turmeric
- sea salt

1 tbsp. Nutritional yeast
½ t. apple cider vinegar
¼ c. of the following:
- water
- raw tahini

4 t. Lemon juice

Follow these simple steps:

1. Set the oven to 350 heat setting.
2. Slice the knobs off the top and bottom of the zucchini, and then slice in half lengthwise.
3. Scoop the center of the seeds from each zucchini with a spoon, creating a bowl to hold the filling.
4. On a big cookie sheet, place the zucchini bowls and bake for approximately 20 minutes.
5. Using a big skillet, combine onion and pepper and sauté for five minutes at medium-high temperature until softened.
6. Add garlic and sauté for an additional minute.
7. Turn the skillet down to medium heat and sprinkle in the chili powder, cumin, salt, and black beans and warm. Remove from the stove and cover to maintain warmth.
8. Prepare the sauce. Using a little bowl, whisk the sauce ingredients until smooth and creamy.
9. Remove the zucchini from the oven when finished cooking.
10. Fill each zucchini bowl generously with the bean mixture.
11. Drizzle the sauce over.
12. Serve warm and enjoy!

Roasted Butternut Squash With Chimichurri

Total Prep & Cooking Time: 30 mins.
Yields: 2 Servings
Nutrition Facts: Calories: 615 | Carbohydrates: 71.6 g | Proteins: 12.5 g | Fats: 35.7 g

Ingredients:
1 c. onion, thinly sliced
2 cloves garlic
1 tbsp. coconut oil
1 acorn squash
2 tbsp. olive oil (best if extra virgin)
¼ c. goji berries
1 c. water
2 c. mushrooms, sliced
½ c. quinoa

Chimichurri Sauce
½ t. salt
2 tbsp. lime
½ c. olive oil, extra virgin
¼ t. cayenne pepper
1 shallot
3 cloves garlic
1 tbsp. sherry vinegar
1 c. parsley

Follow these simple steps:

1. Bring the broiler to the maximum heat setting.
2. Stir up the chimichurri sauce by combining the

parsley, vinegar, garlic shallot, cayenne pepper, olive oil, lime juice, and ½ cup of olive oil. Blend well; if you want the sauce a little thinner, then add additional extra virgin oil.
3. Prepare an aluminum-foiled cookie sheet.
4. Divide the squash in half by carefully cutting widthwise, and remove seeds and pulp from the center.
5. Cut each half of the squash into moon shape slices; you should get about 4-6 slices.
6. Place the slices on the aluminum foil sheet and spritz olive oil across the top.
7. Keep a close eye on the squash; you want nice char marks, nothing more. Once one side is charred to your liking, flip the squash and char the other side.
8. While broiling, bring a medium-sized saucepan of water to a rolling boil then simmer the quinoa, cooking for 10 minutes or until tender.
9. Heat a skillet to medium heat, and sauté the onions. Once the onions are caramelizing, add in the mushroom and garlic, cooking on low heat for approximately 5 minutes.
10. Plate the squash, topping it with quinoa and mushroom.
11. Sprinkle goji berries across the plate and drizzle chimichurri sauce.
12. Serve warm and enjoy!

__Eggplant Pizza__

Total Prep & Cooking Time: 30 mins.
Yields: 8 Servings
Nutrition Facts: Calories: 234 | Carbohydrates: 27 g | Proteins: 5.4 g | Fats: 12 g

Ingredients:
2 tbsp. olive oil
¼ t. of the following:
- pepper
- salt

½ t. oregano, dried
1 c. panko
½ tbsp. almond flour
1 tbsp. flaxseed, ground
1/3 c. water
½ eggplant, medium size
2 c. marinara sauce
1 lb. vegan pizza dough

For the cheese:
¼ lb. tofu, extra firm drained
2 tbsp. almond milk, unsweetened
½ c. cashews, soaked for 6 hours, drained
3 tbsp. lemon juice, freshly squeezed

Follow these simple steps:

1. Set the oven to 400 heat setting; prepare a cookie sheet with ½ tablespoon of olive oil by brushing to

coat.
2. Whisk together flaxseed, flour, and water in a little bowl.
3. In a different bowl, combine salt, pepper, oregano, and panko.
4. Prepare the eggplant by slicing into ¼ inch triangles.
5. Dip each eggplant triangle into the flaxseed mixture then coat with panko mixture and place on the cookie sheet.
6. Slide gently into the oven and baking for 15 minutes. Flip and then bake for an additional 15 minutes or until lightly browned.
7. Take out of the oven and set to the side.
8. Get a pizza stone or pizza pan ready for the dough.
9. Lightly flour the workspace, and with a rolling pin, work the dough to a 14-inch circle then transfer to the pizza stone or pizza pan.
10. Brush the dough's top with olive oil and slide into the warm oven, cooking until lightly browned or for about twenty minutes.
11. While the crust is baking, prepare the cheese by placing cashews in the high-speed blender, blending until it reaches a crumbly consistency.
12. Then add to the blender the lemon juice, almond milk, and tofu; blend until it's a chunky cheese-like consistency. Set to the side.
13. Once the crust is cooked, assemble the pizza by saucing crust with marinara, adding eggplant slices, and placing the cheese on top.
14. Serve warm and enjoy!

Green Avocado Carbonara

Total Prep & Cooking Time: 15 mins.
Yields: 1 Servings
Nutrition Facts: Calories: 526 | Carbohydrates: 24.6 g | Proteins: 5.8 g | Fats: 48.7 g

Ingredients:
Spinach angel hair
Parsley, fresh
2 t. olive oil, extra virgin
2 cloves garlic, diced
½ lemon, zest, and juice
1 avocado, pitted
Salt and pepper to taste

Follow these simple steps:

1. Combine using a food processor the parsley, olive oil, garlic, lemon, and avocado and blend until smooth.
2. Prepare the noodles according to package.
3. Place noodles in a bowl, and add the sauce on top of noodles.
4. Add pepper and salt to your liking.
5. Serve warm and enjoy!

Tofu

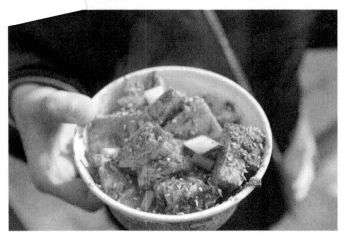

Total Prep & Cooking Time: 30 mins.
Yields: 4 Servings
Nutrition Facts: Calories: 345 | Carbohydrates: 37 g | Proteins: 33.9 g | Fats: 6.3 g

Ingredients:
¼ t. garlic powder
2 tbsp. curry powder
1 pack extra firm tofu

Follow these simple steps:

1. Heat to 400 degrees the oven.
2. Slice the tofu into cubes.
3. In a container with a lid, add the garlic powder, curry powder, and cubed tofu.
4. Close it tightly and shake lightly just to coat the tofu. Make sure there's even coverage of the spices.
5. On a parchment-lined cookie sheet, place the tofu

cubes and bake for 15 minutes, flip and continue baking for another 15 minutes or until crisp.
6. Serve warm and enjoy!

Sesame Tofu and Eggplant

Total Prep & Cooking Time: 20 mins.
Yields: 4 Servings
Nutrition Facts: Calories: 295 | Carbohydrates: 6.87 g | Proteins: 11.21 g | Fats: 6.87 g

Ingredients:
1 tbsp. olive oil
¼ c. of the following:
- sesame seeds
- soy sauce

1 eggplant
1 pound firm tofu
1 t. crushed red pepper flakes
2 cloves garlic
2 t. sweetener of your choice
4 tbsp. toasted sesame oil
1 c. cilantro, chopped
3 tbsp. rice vinegar
Salt and pepper to taste

Follow these simple steps:

1. Set the oven to 200 heat setting.
2. Remove the tofu from the package and blot using paper towels to absorb excess moisture.

3. In a big mixing bowl, whisk together red pepper flakes, garlic, sesame oil, vinegar, and ¼ cup of cilantro to create the marinade.
4. With a mandolin, julienne the eggplant. If you do not have this, you can create the noodles by hand.
5. Mix the noodles in the big bowl with the marinade.
6. Add oil to a skillet over medium-low flame setting, and cook the eggplant until soft.
7. Turn off the oven, and add the last of the cilantro.
8. Transfer the contents from the skillet to an oven-safe dish, cover with foil, and place in the oven to keep warm.
9. Cut the tofu into 8 slices and coat with sesame seeds. Press the sesame seeds into the tofu.
10. In the skillet, add 2 tablespoons of sesame oil and warm under medium heat. Fry the tofu for five minutes then flip and fry.
11. Pour the soy sauce into the pan, coating the tofu. Cook until the tofu looks caramelized.
12. Remove the noodles from the oven and plate with the tofu on top of the noodles.
13. Serve warm and enjoy!

Tempeh Coconut Curry

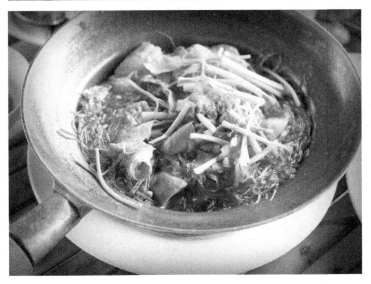

Total Prep & Cooking Time: 30 mins.
Yields: 4 Servings
Nutrition Facts: Calories: 558 | Carbohydrates: 54.2 g | Proteins: 18.4 g | Fats: 33.5 g

Curry:
2 t. of the following:
- low-sodium soy sauce
- tamarind pulp

1 tbsp. of the following:
- lime juice
- garlic, finely chopped
- ginger, finely chopped
- vegetable oil
- salt

8 oz. tempeh

13.5 oz. coconut milk, light
1 c. water
3 c. sweet potato, chopped
1 cinnamon stick
½ t. of the following:
- red pepper, crushed
- turmeric, ground

1 ½ t. coriander, ground
2 c. onion, finely chopped

Rice:
1 ½ c. cauliflower rice
¼ t. salt
1/3 c. cilantro, chopped

Follow these simple steps:

1. Using a medium-high heat setting, warm some oil in a big pot or whatever you prefer, as long as it's nonstick.
2. Place the onion and ½ teaspoon of salt and sauté for approximately 2 minutes.
3. Next, stir in the tamarind, breaking it up as you combine in the skillet and cooking for another 2 minutes.
4. Add in the ginger, garlic, coriander, turmeric, crushed red pepper, and cinnamon stick; stir constantly.
5. Add in the additional salt, tempeh, milk, water, and potatoes, bringing to a boil.
6. Cover, allowing to simmer for fifteen minutes or until tender.

7. Whisk in the soy sauce and simmer for 3 additional minutes.
8. Remove the cinnamon stick.
9. Cook the cauliflower rice according to package instructions.
10. Stir in the cilantro.
11. Place the rice in a bowl and cover with curry.
12. Serve warm and enjoy!

Tempeh Tikka Masala

Total Prep & Cooking Time: 1 h, 35 mins.
Yields: 3 Servings
Nutrition Facts: Calories: 430 | Carbohydrates: 39 g | Proteins: 21 g | Fats: 23 g

Tempeh:
½ t. sea salt
1 t. of the following:
- gram masala
- ginger, ground
- cumin, ground

2 t. apple cider vinegar
½ c. vegan yogurt
8 oz. tempeh, cubed

Tikka Masala Sauce:
2 c. frozen peas
1 c. of the following:
- full-fat coconut milk
- tomato sauce

¼ t. turmeric
½ t. sea salt
1 onion, chopped
1 t. of the following:
- chili powder
- garam masala

1/4 c. ginger, freshly grated
3 cloves garlic, minced
1 tbsp. coconut oil

Follow these simple steps:

1. Begin with making the tempeh by combining sea salt, garam masala, ginger, cumin, vinegar, and yogurt in a bowl.
2. Add tempeh to the bowl and coat well; cover the bowl and refrigerate for 60 minutes.
3. In a pan big enough for 3 servings, add some coconut oil to heat using the medium setting, and begin preparing the sauce.
4. Sauté in the ginger, garlic, and onion for 5 minutes or until fragrant.
5. Add the garam masala, chili powder, sea salt, and turmeric and combine well.
6. Add the frozen peas, coconut, milk, tomato sauce, and tempeh, reducing the heat to medium.
7. Simmer for 15 minutes
8. Remove from the heat and serve with cauliflower rice.

Caprice Casserole

Total Prep & Cooking Time: 1 h, 35 mins.
Yields: 3 Servings
Nutrition Facts: Calories: 642 | Carbohydrates: 88.6 g | Proteins: 25.1 g | Fats: 5.1 g

Tempeh:
¼ c. basil, chopped
1 tomato, big
¼ t. pepper
½ t. salt
1 tbsp. of the following:
- nutritional yeast
- tahini

1 clove garlic
14 oz. tofu, extra firm, drained
6 cups marinara sauce
10 oz. vegetable noodles

Follow these simple steps:

1. Set the oven to 350 heat setting.
2. Cut the tofu into 4 slabs and remove excess moisture by gently squeezing each slab with a paper towel.
3. In a food processor, add garlic and chop, then scrape garlic from the sides to ensure it will be thoroughly mixed.
4. Add pepper, salt, yeast, tahini, and tofu to the food processor and pulse for 15 to 20 seconds until fully combined and forming a paste.

5. In an oven-safe dish, spread ½ cup of the marinara sauce across the bottom.
6. Divide the vegetable noodles in half, break the noodles, and layer them on top of the sauce.
7. Add another layer of sauce on top of the noodles.
8. Add the remaining noodles and coat the top with remaining sauce.
9. Using the tofu mixture from the food processor, form little patties about ½ thick and place on top of the sauce, filling up the dish.
10. Cover the baking container with aluminum foil and bake for 20 minutes.
11. Uncover and bake for an additional fifteen minutes.
12. Remove from the oven and set the oven to broil.
13. Place the tomato slices on top of tofu mixture and broil for 2 minutes or until the tofu is lightly toasted.
14. Garnish with basil.
15. Serve warm and enjoy.

Cheesy Brussel Sprout Bake

Total Prep & Cooking Time: 45 mins.
Yields: 8 Servings
Nutrition Facts: Calories: 116 | Carbohydrates: 16 g | Proteins: 4 g | Fats: 4 g

Ingredients:
½ onion sliced
2 tbsp. of each of these
- garlic, chopped
- avocado oil

1 ½ lb. Brussel sprouts

Cheese:
Dash cayenne
1 t. of the following:
- onion powder
- salt

¼ t. of the following:
- pepper
- paprika

½ t. of the following:
- garlic, powder
- thyme

1 tbsp. tapioca starch
¼ c. nutritional yeast
½ c. vegetable broth
1 can coconut cream

Crumble Topping :

¼ t. pepper
½ t. garlic, powder
1 t. salt
½ c. panko crumbs

Follow these simple steps:

1. Bring the oven to 425 heat setting.
2. Prepare Brussel sprouts by washing and trimming then steaming for 10 minutes.
3. Spray an oven-safe baking dish with nonstick spray.
4. Add the Brussel sprouts to a baking dish and set to the side.
5. Bring a skillet to medium temperature and mix in the garlic, avocado oil, and onion, sautéing approximately 6 minutes.
6. Add the onion mixture to the top of the Brussel sprouts.
7. In the same skillet on low heat, add vegetable broth, nutritional yeast, onion powder, pepper, salt, garlic, paprika, thyme, and coconut cream, whisking together to combine.
8. Carefully add in the tapioca starch and whisk constantly; the mixture will thicken in about 5 minutes. Once it turns into a cheese sauce mixture, pour over the Brussel sprouts and onions.
9. In a mixing container, combine panko, salt, garlic, and pepper, creating the crumble.
10. Sprinkle the crumble across the top of the cheese.
11. Cook in the oven for approximately 25 minutes or until browned and golden.

12. Serve warm and enjoy.

Tofu Noodle Bowl

Total Prep & Cooking Time: 45 mins.
Yields: 4 Servings
Nutrition Facts: Calories: 669 | Carbohydrates: 69 g | Proteins: 55.1 g | Fats: 24.7g

Ingredients:
¼ c. of the following
- peanuts, chopped
- cilantro, chopped

4 heads baby bok choy, chopped
2 packages premade baked tofu, 8 oz.
½ t. black pepper, ground
2 t. of the following:
- turmeric, ground
- garlic chili sauce

1 tbsp. of the following:
- lime juice
- ginger, minced

2 c. vegetable stock
2 carrots, julienned
1 red bell pepper, chopped
½ red onion, diced
2 cloves garlic, minced
1 t. peanut oil
6 oz. Thai rice noodles

Follow these simple steps:

1. Prepare the Thai noodles, following the package guidelines or according to your preference.
2. Warm a big pan using medium-high heat, adding in the peanut oil.
3. Sauté the ginger, garlic, and onion for approximately 5 minutes.
4. Next, add in the carrots and bell pepper, stirring frequently and cooking for 5 minutes.
5. Whisk together the lime juice, black pepper, turmeric, chili sauce, and stock, then combine with the pan of peppers and carrots.
6. Wait for the mixture to boil, and soon after, bring down the heat setting, and leave it cooking for nearly 5 minutes.
7. As it simmers, add in the noodles, bok choy, and tofu and cook for an additional 5 minutes.
8. Divide between bowls and garnish with chili peppers, peanuts, and cilantro.
9. Serve warm and enjoy.

Cashew Siam Salad

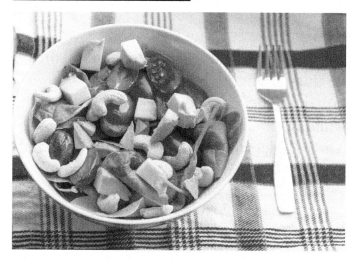

Total Prep & Cooking Time: 25 mins.
Yields: 4 Servings
Nutrition Facts: Calories: 352 | Carbohydrates: 26.6 g | Proteins: 9.6 g | Fats: 24.5 g

Ingredients:
3 green onions, chopped
2/3 c. sunflower seeds
1 bag slaw mix
2 packages ramen noodles
1 c. cashews, crushed
1 t. olive oil

Dressing:
Seasoning packets from ramen noodles
1 c. vinegar
½ c. sweetener of your choice

Follow these simple steps:

1. Set the oven to 350 heat setting.
2. In a mixing container, combine cashews and oil and mix until the nuts are lightly oiled.
3. Place the nuts on a lined cookie sheet and toast until lightly browned in the oven.
4. In a big mixing bowl, crumble the ramen noodles and combine with slaw mix, sunflower seeds, and green onion.
5. Whisk together the vinegar and sweetener of your choice in a little bowl until combined.
6. Remove the peanuts from the oven and cool.
7. Place the salad in a bowl and cover the top with peanuts.
8. When ready to serve, add the dressing, and enjoy.

Cucumber Edamame Salad

Total Prep & Cooking Time: 2 hours mins.
Yields: 8 Servings
Nutrition Facts: Calories: 166 | Carbohydrates: 6.4 g | Proteins: 2.9 g | Fats: 14.9 g

Ingredients:
1 jalapeno pepper, seeded and chopped
2 c. froze edamame, shelled and thawed
4 English cucumbers, spiralizer

Vinaigrette:
1 t. red pepper flakes
1 ½ t. of the following:
- garlic
- Dijon mustard
- soy sauce, low-sodium

2 t. ginger, paste
3 t. toasted sesame oil
1/3 c. of the following:
- rice vinegar
- extra virgin olive oil

Follow these simple steps:

1. Begin by cleaning your cucumbers and spiraling them to create the noodles.
2. Once cucumbers are spiraled, use a towel or cheesecloth to discard the excess moisture out of the noodles.

3. In a big mixing bowl, add noodles, jalapeno, red bell pepper, and edamame. Carefully toss the salad mixture and set to the side.
4. In a little mixing container, prepare the vinaigrette by whisking together the red pepper flakes, garlic, Dejon, soy sauce, ginger, oil, rice vinegar, and olive oil.
5. Lightly coat the salad with dressing.
6. Cover and refrigerate overnight or a minimum of 2 hours.
7. Serve cool and enjoy.

Caesar Vegan Salad

Total Prep & Cooking Time: 30 mins.
Yields: 6 Servings
Nutrition Facts: Calories: 284 | Carbohydrates: 25.5 g | Proteins: 8.7 g | Fats: 18.4 g

Ingredients:
5 c. kale, chopped
10 c. romaine lettuce

Cheese:
½ t. garlic
1 tbsp. of the following:
- extra virgin olive oil
- nutritional yeast

1 garlic clove
2 tbsp. hemp seeds, hulled
1/3 c. cashews, raw

Caesar Dressing:
½ t. of the following:
- sea salt
- garlic powder
- Dijon mustard

2 t. capers
½ tbsp. vegan Worcestershire sauce
2 tbsp. olive oil (best if extra virgin)
½ c. raw cashews, soaked overnight
¼ c. water
1 clove garlic, crushed
1 tbsp. lemon juice

Croutons:
1/8 t. cayenne pepper
½ t. of the following:
- garlic powder
- sea salt

1 t. olive oil, (best if extra virgin)
14 oz. can chickpeas

Follow these simple steps:

1. On the day before you plan to make this salad, in a little bowl, soak ½ c. of the raw cashews overnight then drain and rinse.
2. For the Croutons – Bring the oven to 400 heat setting. Drain the chickpeas and rinse thoroughly. Using a tea towel or cheesecloth, rub the chickpeas so that the skins fall off. Place those in a dish for baking. Spritz the chickpeas with oil and roll them around to

coat. Season with cayenne, salt, and garlic powder. Roast the chickpeas for approximately a quarter of an hour or until you are satisfied with the color. Remove from the oven, allowing to cool and become firm.
3. For the Dressing – Combine everything but not the salt, either in a processor or blender. Blend until smooth liquid consistency. If needed, add ½ tablespoon of water at a time until you have a dressing-like consistency. Season with salt to taste. Set to the side.
4. For the Cheese – In a food processor, add garlic and cashews and process them until they reach a finely chopped consistency. Add hemp seeds, nutritional yeast, olive oil, and garlic powder and blend until combined. Season with salt to taste.
5. For the lettuce – After washing the kale, finely chop and set to the side. Chop the lettuce roughly into 2-inch pieces and toss with the kale in a bowl.
6. Pour some dressing and toss again to coat the greens fully.
7. Sprinkle the cheese and croutons over the top.
8. Serve cool and enjoy.

Mushroom Lettuce Wraps

Total Prep & Cooking Time: 30 mins.
Yields: 4 Servings
Nutrition Facts: Calories: 265 | Carbohydrates: 37.6 g | Proteins: 13.6 g | Fats: 7.9 g

Ingredients:
8 big leaf romaine lettuce
4 green onions, sliced
¼ t. red pepper flakes
2 t. of the following:
- ginger, grated
- canola oil

2 cloves garlic
12 oz. extra firm tofu
1 t. sesame oil
2 tbsp. rice vinegar
8 oz. mushrooms, diced
1 can water chestnuts
3 tbsp. of the following:
- soy sauce, reduced-sodium
- hoisin Sauce

Follow these simple steps:

1. Whisk together in a little bowl the sesame oil, rice vinegar, soy sauce, and hoisin. Then set to the side.
2. Open the tofu, and using a paper towel or cheesecloth, remove as much liquid as you can.
3. In a big skillet over medium-high heat, warm the 2

teaspoons of canola oil.
4. Crumble the tofu, making it into little pieces and cook for approximately 5 minutes.
5. Add in the diced mushrooms and cook until almost all the liquid evaporates.
6. Add in the green onions, red pepper, ginger, garlic, and chestnuts and cook for about 30 seconds.
7. Pour the sauce from the little bowl into the skillet and cook until sauce is thoroughly warmed.
8. Plate the individual lettuce leaves and spoon the tofu mixture into each lettuce wrap.
9. Serve and enjoy warm.

Chapter 6: Side Dishes & Snacks

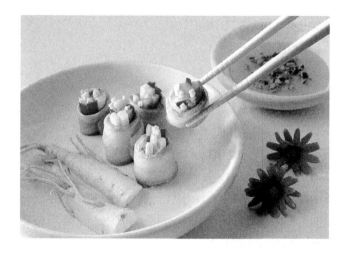

For those special occasions, just prepare a tasty snack or a beautiful side dish.

Mixed Seed Crackers

Total Prep & Cooking Time: 60 min.
Yields: 30 Servings
Nutrition Facts: Calories: 61 | Carbohydrates: 1 g | Proteins: 2 g | Fats: 6 g

Ingredients:

1 c. boiling water
¼ c. coconut oil, melted
1 t. salt
1 tbsp. psyllium husk powder

1/3 c. of the following:
- sesame seeds
- flaxseed
- pumpkin seeds, unsalted
- sunflower seeds, unsalted
- almond flour

Follow these simple steps:

1. Set the oven to 300 setting.
2. With a fork, combine the almond flour, seeds, psyllium, and salt.
3. Cautiously pour the boiling water and oil to the bowl, using the fork to combine.
4. The mixture should form a gel-like consistency.
5. Line a cookie sheet using a non-stick paper or a similar alternative, and transfer the mixture to the cookie sheet.
6. Using the second sheet of parchment, place it on top of the mixture, and with a rolling pin, roll out the mixture to an even and flat consistency.
7. Remove the top parchment paper and bake in the oven for 40 minutes, checking frequently to ensure the seeds do not burn.
8. After 40 minutes, or when the seeds are browning, turn off the oven but leave the crackers inside for further cooking.
9. Once cool break into pieces and enjoy

Crispy Squash Chips

Total Prep & Cooking Time: 30 min.
Yields: 2 Servings
Nutrition Facts: Calories: 83 | Carbohydrates: 5.8 g | Proteins: 0.5 g | Fats: 7 g

Ingredients:

1 t. cayenne pepper
1 t. cumin
1 t. paprika
1 tbsp. avocado oil
1 medium butternut squash, skinny neck
Sea salt to taste

Follow these simple steps:

1. Set the oven to 375 heat setting.
2. Prepare the butternut squash by removing the top.
3. Using a mandolin, cut the squash into even slices; it is not necessary to skin the squash.
4. In a big mixing bowl, place your slices of squash and cover with oil, using your hands to mix them well. Ensure all slices are oiled.
5. Line a cookie sheet with parchment paper and spread out your slices, so they do not overlap.
6. In a little bowl, mix together cayenne pepper, paprika, and cumin then sprinkle the chips over the top.
7. Season with sea salt to taste
8. Once cool, enjoy alone or with your favorite dip.

Paprika Nuts

Total Prep & Cooking Time: 30 min.
Yields: 8 Servings
Nutrition Facts: Calories: 417 | Carbohydrates: 12.4 g | Proteins: 10.8 g | Fats: 39.2 g

Ingredients:

1 ½ t. smoked paprika
1 t. salt
2 tbsp. garlic-infused olive oil
1 c. of the following:
- cashews
- almonds
- pecans
- walnuts

Follow these simple steps:

1. Adjust the racks in the oven so that there is one rack in the middle.
2. Set the oven to 325 before you start preparing the ingredients.
3. In a big mixing bowl, toss the nuts.
4. Pour olive oil over the nuts and toss to coat all the nuts.
5. Sprinkle the salt and paprika over the nuts and mix well. If you want more paprika flavor, then add additional paprika.
6. Line a big cookie sheet with parchment and spread the nuts out in one layer.

7. Bake for approximately 15 minutes, then remove from oven and let cool.
8. Enjoy.

Basil Zoodles and Olives

Total Prep & Cooking Time: 4 hr. 30 min.
Yields: 6 Servings
Nutrition Facts: Calories: 117 | Carbohydrates: 9.8 g | Proteins: 3.5 g | Fats: 8.4 g

Ingredients:

1 can black olives pitted
1 little container cherry tomatoes, halved
4 medium-size zucchini

Sauce:

½ c basil leaves, chopped
½ t. pink Himalayan salt
2 t. nutritional yeast
1 tbsp. lemon juice
½ c. water
¼ c. of the following:
- sunflower seeds, soaked
- cashew nuts, soaked

Follow these simple steps:

1. Begin by preparing the sunflower seeds and cashews. Place each in a little bowl and cover with water. Allow to soak for 4 hours then drain and rinse well.
2. Next, place the seeds and cashews into a blender and mix until completely blended. Then add in basil, salt, nutritional yeast, lemon juice, and water. Blend until a smooth sauce is formed.
3. Using a spiralizer, make the zoodles from the zucchini.
4. Place the zoodles in a big serving bowl and then pour the sauce over the top. Stir to combine.
5. Top with cherry tomatoes and olives.
6. Serve and enjoy.

Roasted Beetroot Noodles

Total Prep & Cooking Time: 35 min.
Yields: 4 Servings
Nutrition Facts: Calories: 79 | Carbohydrates: 4.1 g | Proteins: 1 g | Fats: 7 g

Ingredients:

1 t. orange zest
2 tbsp. of the following:
- parsley, chopped
- balsamic vinegar
- olive oil

2 big beets, peeled and spiraled

Follow these simple steps:

1. Set the oven to 425 high-heat setting.
2. In a big bowl, combine the beet noodles, olive oil, and vinegar. Toss until well-combined. Season with salt and pepper to your liking.
3. Line a big cookie sheet with parchment paper, and spread the noodles out into a single layer. Roast the noodles for 20 minutes.
4. Place into bowls and zest with orange and sprinkle parsley. Gently toss and serve.

Turnip Fries

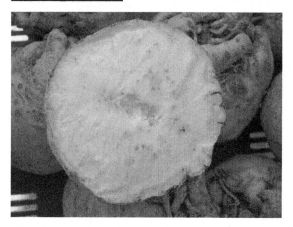

Total Prep & Cooking Time: 45 min.
Yields: 4 Servings
Nutrition Facts: Calories: 83 | Carbohydrates: 11.6 g | Proteins: 3.2 g | Fats: 3.1 g

Ingredients:

1 t. of the following:
- onion powder
- paprika
- garlic salt

1 tbsp. vegetable oil
3 pounds turnips

Follow these simple steps:

1. Set the oven to 425 heat setting.
2. Prepare a lightly greased aluminum foil-lined cookie sheet

3. Using a hand peeler, peel the turnips. With a Mandolin, cut the turnips into French fry sticks. Then place in a big bowl.
4. Toss the turnips with oil to coat then season with onion powder, paprika, and garlic and coat again.
5. Spread evenly across the cookie sheet.
6. Bake for 20 minutes or until the outside is crisp.
7. Serve with your favorite sauce or enjoy alone.

Lime and Chili Carrots Noodles

Total Prep & Cooking Time: 10 min.
Yields: 4 Servings
Nutrition Facts: Calories: 89 | Carbohydrates: 7 g | Proteins: 1 g | Fats: 7 g

Ingredients:

½ t. of the following:
- black pepper
- salt

2 tbsp. coconut oil
¼ c. coriander, finely chopped
2 Jalapeno chili's
1 tbsp. lime juice
2 carrots, peeled and spiralized

Follow these simple steps:

1. In a little bowl, combine jalapeno, lime juice, and coconut oil to form a sauce.
2. In a big bowl, place the carrot noodles and pour dressing over the top.
3. Toss to ensure the dressing fully coats the noodles.
4. Season with salt and pepper to your liking.
5. Serve and enjoy.

Pesto Zucchini Noodles

Total Prep & Cooking Time: 15 min.
Yields: Servings
Nutrition Facts: Calories: 166 | Carbohydrates: 4.5g | Proteins: 1.6 g | Fats: 17 g

Ingredients:

4 little zucchini ends trimmed
Cherry tomatoes
2 t. fresh lemon juice
1/3 c olive oil (best if extra-virgin)
2 cups packed basil leaves
2 c. garlic
Salt and pepper to taste

Follow these simple steps:

1. Spiral zucchini into noodles and set to the side.
2. In a food processor, combine the basil and garlic and chop. Slowly add olive oil while chopping. Then pulse blend it until thoroughly mixed.
3. In a big bowl, place the noodles and pour pesto sauce over the top. Toss to combine.
4. Garnish with tomatoes and serve and enjoy.

Cabbage Slaw

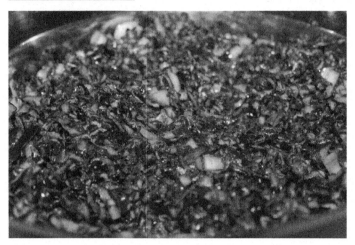

Total Prep & Cooking Time: 5 min.
Yields: 6 Servings
Nutrition Facts: Calories: 276 | Carbohydrates: 11.7 g | Proteins: 0 g | Fats: 9.3 g

Ingredients:

1/8 t. celery seed
¼ t. salt
2 tbsp. of the following:
- apple cider vinegar
- sweetener of your choice

½ c. vegan mayo
4 c. coleslaw mix with red cabbage and carrots

Follow these simple steps:

1. In a big mixing bowl, whisk together the celery seed, salt, apple cider vinegar, sweetener, and vegan mayo.

2. Add the coleslaw and stir until appropriately combined.
3. Refrigerate while covered for a minimum of 2 hours or overnight if you're not in a hurry.
4. Garnish with tomatoes and serve and enjoy.

Zucchini Chips

Total Prep & Cooking Time: 1 hr. 40 min
Yields: 4 Servings
Nutrition Facts: Calories: 276 | Carbohydrates: 11.7 g | Proteins: 0 g | Fats: 9.3 g

Ingredients:

2 tbsp. olive oil (best if extra virgin)
1 big zucchini
½ t. of the following:
- black pepper, ground
- salt

Follow these simple steps:

1. Bring the oven to 400 heat setting.
2. Using a mandolin, slice the zucchini into $1/8^{th}$-inch slices.
3. Once sliced, use a paper towel to remove the excess moisture from the zucchini by blotting the tops.
4. Prepare two cookie sheets with parchment paper, and spread the zucchini out into a single layer.

5. Whisk well the olive oil and seasonings. With this mixture, brush each zucchini.
6. Bake this for 60 minutes then flip.
7. Check every 20 minutes, and once the zucchini is crispy, remove from the oven and serve.

Peanut Tofu Wrap

Total Prep & Cooking Time: 30 min
Yields: 4 Servings
Nutrition Facts: Calories: 186 | Carbohydrates: 8 g | Proteins: 13 g | Fats: 12 g

Ingredients:
¼ c. cilantro, finely chopped
1 c. of the following:
- Asian pear
- English cucumber

1 ½ t. lime zest
1 tbsp. of the following:
- rice vinegar
- canola oil

5 tbsp. peanut sauce
14 oz. tofu, extra firm
8 cabbage leaves

Follow these simple steps:

1. Prepare cabbage leaves by washing and drying. Be sure to remove any stems or ribs.
2. Place the tofu on a paper towel-lined plate and blot to remove the extra moisture.
3. Set a big nonstick skillet over medium-high heat and place the oil. Once the oil is warm, add the tofu and crumble it to cook, stirring often. Wait for approximately 5 minutes or until the tofu turns golden brown. Remove from the heat and set to the side.

4. Mix well using a spatula the liquid ingredients, except the oil, and add the lime zest.
5. Add the sauce to the skillet and combine.
6. Place the cabbage leaves on the plates and spoon the tofu mixture into the center, topping it with cilantro, cucumber, and pear.

Cinnamon Granola

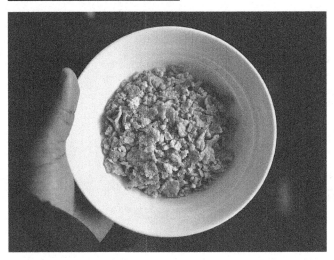

Total Prep & Cooking Time: 25 min
Yields: 4 Servings
Nutrition Facts: Calories: 175 | Carbohydrates: 11 g | Proteins: 6 g | Fats: 17 g

Ingredients:
1 ½ t. cinnamon, ground
4 tbsp. maple syrup
1/5 oz. nuts
1 tbsp. chia seeds

5 tbsp. of the following:
- coconut flakes, unsweetened
- flaxseed meal

Follow these simple steps:
1. Bring the oven to 350 heat setting.
2. In a medium mixing bowl, combine the flaxseed, coconut, chia seed, nuts, and maple syrup. Mix well until combined.
3. Line a cookie sheet with parchment and spread the mixture in a single layer on the cookie sheet.
4. Across the top, sprinkle the cinnamon.
5. Place the cookie sheet in the oven, and wait for 20 minutes, approximately.
6. Once done, take it out and allow the granola to cool while still on the sheet.
7. Once cool, crumble to your desired liking and enjoy.

Chocolate Granola

Total Prep & Cooking Time: 60 min
Yields: 12 Servings
Nutrition Facts: Calories: 302 | Carbohydrates: 5.6 g | Proteins: 9.7 g | Fats: 24.8 g

Ingredients:
¼ t. sea salt
¼ c. of the following:
- hot water
- cocoa powder

1/3 c. of the following:
- coconut oil
- maple syrup, sugar-free

½ c. of the following:
- almond butter
- almond flour
- cashews, chopped

1 c. mixed seeds (flaxseed, sesame, sunflower, pumpkin)
2 c. coconut, flaked
2/3 c. almonds, flaked

Follow these simple steps:

1. Bring the oven to 300 heat setting.
2. In a little bowl, mix cocoa and hot water to form a thick paste.
3. Next, add to the little bowl the coconut oil, maple syrup, nut butter, and salt; mix until combined thoroughly.

4. In a big bowl, mix the almond meal, coconut flakes, seeds, and nuts.
5. Transfer the chocolate mixture to the big bowl and combine well.
6. Using a parchment-lined cookie sheet, spread out the granola mixture.
7. Bake for 40 minutes or until firm.
8. Allow to completely cool on the parchment.
9. Once cool, crumble to your desired liking and enjoy.

Radish Chips

Total Prep & Cooking Time: 1 hr. 40 min
Yields: 4 Servings
Nutrition Facts: Calories: 70 | Carbohydrates: 2.2 g | Proteins: 0.4 g | Fats: 7.1 g

Ingredients:

2 tbsp. olive oil (best if extra virgin)
16 oz. radishes
½ t. of the following:
- Black pepper, ground
- Salt

Follow these simple steps:

1. Bring the oven to 400 heat setting.
2. Using a mandolin, slice the radishes into 1/8th-inch slices.

3. Once sliced, use a paper towel to remove the excess moisture from the radishes by blotting the tops.
4. Prepare two cookie sheets with parchment paper, and spread the zucchini out into a single layer.
5. Add the seasonings in a bowl, with the olive oil. Whisk well and then brush each radish with this mixture, coating evenly and generously.
6. Bake for 10 minutes and then flip
7. Check every 5 minutes; once the radish is crispy, remove from the oven and serve.

Asparagus Fries

Total Prep & Cooking Time: 1 hr. 35 min
Yields: 4 Servings
Nutrition Facts: Calories: 183 | Carbohydrates: 10 g | Proteins: 8 g | Fats: 14 g

Ingredients:

2 tbsp. nutritional yeast
1 c. almond meal
1 t. of the following:
- maple syrup
- smoked paprika
- Himalayan pink salt

½ t. black pepper, ground
1 t. extra virgin olive oil
1 bunch asparagus

Follow these simple steps:

1. Set the oven to 400.
2. Prepare the asparagus by washing and cutting into equal halves.
3. In a big bowl, place the asparagus, add olive oil to the top, and toss to coat.
4. Add to the bowl the syrup, paprika, pepper, and salt and toss to coat.
5. In a medium, shallow bowl, mix the almond meal and nutritional yeast.
6. Line a cookie sheet with parchment paper and set to the side
7. Individually add each asparagus piece to the bowl, coating with your crumb mixture.
8. Place the asparagus on a lined cookie sheet; be sure not to overlap them.
9. Bake for 20 minutes or until brown.
10. Remove from the oven and serve.

Chapter 7: Sauces & Dips

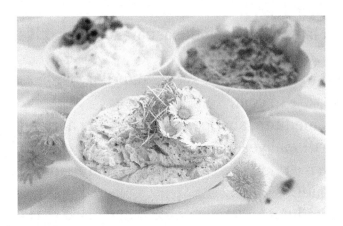

Keto-Vegan Ketchup

Total Prep & Cooking Time: 35 min.
Yields: 12 Servings
Nutrition Facts: Calories: 13 | Carbohydrates: 2 g | Proteins: 0 g | Fats: 0 g

Ingredients:

1/8 t of the following:
- mustard powder
- cloves, ground

¼ t. paprika
½ t. garlic powder
¾ t. onion powder
1 t. sea salt
3 tbsp. apple cider vinegar
¼ c. powdered monk fruit
1 c. water

6 oz. tomato paste

Follow these simple steps:

1. In a little saucepan, whisk together all the ingredients.
2. Cover the pan and bring to low heat and simmer for 30 minutes, stirring occasionally.
3. Once reduced, add to the blender and puree until it's a smooth consistency.
4. Enjoy.

Avocado Hummus

Total Prep & Cooking Time: 5 min.
Yields: 6 Servings
Nutrition Facts: Calories: 310 | Carbohydrates: 26 g | Proteins: 8 g | Fats: 20 g

Ingredients:

1 tbsp. cilantro, finely chopped
1/8 t. cumin
1 clove garlic
3 tbsp. lime juice
1 ½ tbsp. of the following:
- tahini
- olive oil

2 avocados, medium cored & peeled
15 oz. chickpeas, drained
Salt and pepper to taste

Follow these simple steps:

1. In a food processor, add garlic, lime juice, tahini, olive oil, and chickpeas and pulse until combined.
2. Add cumin and avocados and blend until smooth consistency approximately 2 minutes.
3. Add salt and pepper to taste.
4. Enjoy.

Guacamole

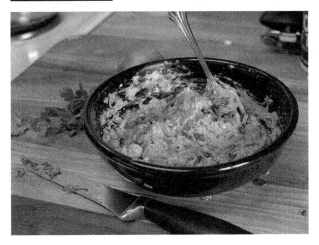

Total Prep & Cooking Time: 5 min.
Yields: 6 Servings
Nutrition Facts: Calories: 127 | Carbohydrates: 9.3 g | Proteins: 2.4 g | Fats: 10.2 g

Ingredients:

3 tbsp. of the following:
- tomato, diced
- onion, diced

2 tbsp. of the following:
- cilantro, chopped
- jalapeno juice

¼ t. garlic powder
½ t. salt
½ lime, squeezed
2 big avocados
1 jalapeno, diced

Follow these simple steps:

1. Using a molcajete, crush the diced jalapenos until soft.
2. Add the avocados to the molcajete.
3. Squeeze the lime juice from ½ of the lime on top of the avocados.
4. Add the jalapeno juice, garlic, and salt and mix until smooth.
5. Once smooth, add in the onion, cilantro, and tomato and stir to incorporate.
6. Enjoy.

Keto-Vegan Mayo

Total Prep & Cooking Time: 5 min.
Yields: 6 Servings
Nutrition Facts: Calories: 160.4 | Carbohydrates: 0.2 g | Proteins: 0 g | Fats: 18 g

Ingredients:

½ c. of the following:
- extra virgin olive oil
- almond milk, unsweetened

¼ t. xanthan gum
Pinch of white pepper, ground
Pinch of Himalayan salt
1 t. Dijon mustard
2 t. apple cider vinegar

Follow these simple steps:

1. In a blender, place milk, pepper salt, mustard, and vinegar.
2. Turn the blender to high speed and slowly add xanthan then the olive oil.
3. Remove from the blender and allow cooling for 2 hours in the refrigerator.
4. During cooling, the mixture will thicken.

uce

Prep & Cooking Time: 10 min.
Yields: 4 Servings
Nutrition Facts: Calories: 151 | Carbohydrates: 4 g | Proteins: 4 g | Fats: 13 g

Ingredients:

½ t. Thai red curry paste
1 t. of the following:
- coconut oil
- soy Sauce
- chili garlic sauce

1 tbsp. sweetener of your choice
1/3 c. coconut milk
1.4 c. peanut butter, smooth

Follow these simple steps:

1. Using a microwave-safe dish, add the peanut butter and heat for about 30 seconds.
2. Whisk into the peanut butter, the soy sauce, sweetener, and chili garlic then set to the side.
3. Warm a little saucepan over medium heat and add oil.
4. Cook the Thai red curry paste until fragrant then add to a microwave-safe bowl.
5. Continuously stir the peanut mixture as you add the coconut milk. Stir until well-combined.
6. Enjoy at room temperature or warmed.

Pistachio Dip

Total Prep & Cooking Time: 10 min.
Yields: 8 Servings
Nutrition Facts: Calories: 88 | Carbohydrates: 9 g | Proteins: 2.5 g | Fats: 3 g

Ingredients:

2 tbsp. lemon juice
1 t. extra virgin olive oil
2 tbsp. of the following:
- tahini
- parsley, chopped

2 cloves of garlic
½ c. pistachios shelled
15 oz. garbanzo beans, save the liquid from the can
Salt and pepper to taste

Follow these simple steps:

1. Using a food processor, add pistachios, pepper, sea salt, lemon juice, olive oil, tahini, parsley, garlic, and garbanzo beans. Pulse until mixed.
2. Using the liquid from the garbanzo beans, add to the dip while slowly blending until it reaches your desired consistency.
3. Enjoy at room temperature or warmed.

Smokey Tomato Jam

Total Prep & Cooking Time: 45 min.
Yields: 1 Cup
Nutrition Facts: Calories: 26 | Carbohydrates: 5.3 g | Proteins: 1.1 g | Fats: 0.6 g

Ingredients:

½ t. of the following:
- white wine vinegar
- salt

1/3 t. smoked paprika
Pinch Black pepper
¼ c. coconut sugar
2 pounds tomatoes

Follow these simple steps:

1. Over medium-high heat, bring a big pot of water to a boil.
2. Fill a big bowl with ice and water.
3. Carefully place the tomatoes into the boiling water for 1 minute and then remove, and immediately put into the ice water.
4. While tomatoes are in the ice water, peel them by hand and then transfer to a clean cutting surface.
5. Empty the pot of water.
6. Chop the tomatoes and place back into the pot; add in the coconut sugar and stir to combine.
7. Bring the pot back to medium heat and the tomatoes to a boil, cooking for 15 minutes.

8. Stir in the paprika, pepper, and salt and then bring the temperature down to the lowest setting. Let it cook until it becomes thick, which is approximately 10 minutes.
9. Remove it from the heat while continuing to stir; add in white wine vinegar.

Tasty Ranch Dressing/Dip

Total Prep & Cooking Time: 45 min.
Yields: 16 servings
Nutrition Facts: Calories: 93 | Carbohydrates: 0 g | Proteins: 0 g | Fats: 9 g

Ingredients:

½ c. soy milk, unsweetened
1 tbsp. dill, chopped
2 t. parsley, chopped
¼ t. black pepper
½ t. of the following:
- onion powder
- garlic powder

1 c. vegan mayonnaise

Follow these simple steps:

1. In a medium bowl, whisk all the ingredients together until smooth. If dressing is too thick, add ¼ tablespoon of soy milk at a time until the desired consistency.

2. Transfer to an airtight container or jar and refrigerate for 1 hour.
3. Serve over leafy greens or as a dip.

Chapter 8: Soups

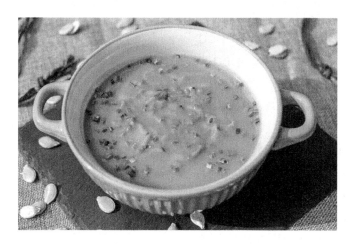

These recipes are for those days when a hearty warm soup just hits the spot.

Goulash Soup

Total Prep & Cooking Time: 35 min.
Yields: 7 Servings
Nutrition Facts: Calories: 267 | Carbohydrates: 51.7 g | Proteins: 11.7 g | Fats: 3.1 g

Ingredients:

½ t. black pepper
14.5 oz. tomatoes, diced
8 little rutabagas, chopped into ½ inch chunks
¼ c. dry red wine
4 tbsp. paprika

1 t. salt
3 c. vegetable broth
6 cloves of garlic, minced
2 red bell peppers, chopped
2 c. onion, finely chopped

Follow these simple steps:

1. Prior to starting, ensure that you have all the vegetables washed and chopped. This recipe moves very quickly.
2. In a pot that is big enough for 7 servings, add the onion, garlic, and bell pepper after it has warmed in a medium heat setting.
3. Add to the pot ½ teaspoon of salt and 1 cup of the broth. Wait for it to bubble and then leave it cooking until the broth is gone. This usually just takes about 8 minutes.
4. Lower the temperature, and add the wine when most of the broth has evaporated. Add the paprika. Let the flavor seep in for a couple of minutes or a bit more.
5. Next, add the rest of the salt, pepper, tomatoes, rutabagas, and 1 ½ cup of broth. If you would like your dish to become saucier, add in the additional broth. Cook for 20 minutes or until the rutabaga is tender.
6. Serve and enjoy!

Celery Dill Soup

Total Prep & Cooking Time: 35 min.
Yields: 4 Servings
Nutrition Facts: Calories: 176 | Carbohydrates: 30.2 g | Proteins: 5.6 g | Fats: 13.6 g

Ingredients:

3 t. olive oil
½ c. pickle juice
½ onion, chopped
½ t. xanthan gum
¼ c dill pickle, finely chopped
1 stalk celery, chopped
¼ c. vegetable broth
1 t. of the following:
- parsley
- garlic, minced

1 tbsp. ghee
½ c. vegan bacon, crumbled

Follow these simple steps:

1. Before beginning, ensure you have chopped all vegetables.
2. In a big saucepan, melt ghee and garlic.
3. Add in the chopped pickles, onion, celery, and parsley and sauté for 5 minutes.
4. Next, add vegetable broth and pickle juice and bring to a boil.

5. In a little bowl, whisk together xanthan gum and olive oil then pour into the soup.
6. Continue to stir the soup frequently as it thickens.
7. Once thick, add crumbled bacon and serve.

Broccoli Fennel Soup

Total Prep & Cooking Time: 35 min.
Yields: 4 Servings
Nutrition Facts: Calories: 242 | Carbohydrates: 23.2 g | Proteins: 7.6 g | Fats: 15.4 g

Ingredients:

2 ½ c. kale
2 tbsp. lemon juice
3 c. water
½ c. cashews
1 medium onion, chopped
5 cloves garlic, minced
2 tbsp. olive oil
2 c. fennel, chopped
4 c. broccoli florets

Follow these simple steps:

1. Bring the oven to 400 heat setting.
2. Prepare a cookie sheet by lining it with paper.
3. Spread the florets and fennel on the cookie sheet; be careful not to overlap them and drizzle with 1 tablespoon of olive oil.

4. Place in the oven and roast for 10 minutes then flip and roast for another 10 minutes.
5. While it is roasting, bring a heat a saucepan over medium-low heat.
6. Add in the remaining olive oil, and sauté the garlic for about 3 minutes; add in the onion and sauté for an additional 3 minutes.
7. After broccoli and fennel are finished roasting, add to the pan with the onion and garlic; mix thoroughly.
8. Finally, add the kale, lemon juice, water, and cashews. Simmer this for approximately 5 minutes.
9. Remove it from the stove and then blend using a machine you prefer, as long as it gets smooth.
10. Dust some salt and pepper or not, if you don't like additional salt. Serve.

Broccoli and Cauliflower Soup

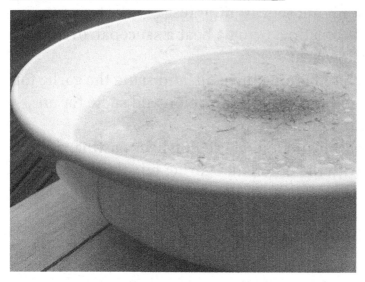

Total Prep & Cooking Time: 35 min.
Yields: 8 Servings
Nutrition Facts: Calories: 204 | Carbohydrates: 14.7 g | Proteins: 9.5 g | Fats: 13.6 g

Ingredients:

1 tbsp. lemon juice
1 ½ t. salt
1/3 c. nutritional yeast
1 c. almond milk, unsweetened
4 c. vegetable broth
¼ c. almond flour
4 c. cauliflower, finely chopped
4 c. broccoli, finely chopped
2 carrots, diced
2 cloves garlic, minced

1 onion, chopped
2 tbsp. extra virgin olive oil

Follow these simple steps:

1. Pour some olive oil to a big-enough saucepan that has warmed using the medium heat setting.
2. Sauté for more than a couple of minutes the garlic, onion, and seasonings.
3. Add the chopped veggies (carrots, cauliflower, and broccoli) and sauté for another 5 minutes.
4. Next, add in the flour and stir to combine.
5. Once combined, add in the nutritional yeast, milk, and broth and then wait for it to boil just before turning the heat setting to medium-low.
6. While covered, let it simmer for about a quarter of an hour or less. Stir once in a while as you wait.
7. Remove from the heat and add in lemon juice. Using a hand blender, blend the soup contents until your desired level of chunkiness.
8. Dust with some salt and pepper to your taste and serve.

Keto-Vegan Chili

Total Prep & Cooking Time: 41 min.
Yields: 6 Servings
Nutrition Facts: Calories: 294 | Carbohydrates: 17.1 g | Proteins: 10.6 g | Fats: 23.7 g

Ingredients:

1 tbsp. cocoa powder, unsweetened
1 c. raw walnuts
16 oz. tofu, extra firm
½ c. coconut milk
3 c. water
15 oz. diced tomatoes
1 ½ tbsp. tomato paste
8 oz. cremini mushrooms
2 zucchini, diced
2 green bell peppers, diced
2 chipotle peppers in adobo sauce, minced
1 ½ t. paprika
4 t. cumin
2 t. chili powder
1 ½ t. cinnamon, ground
2 cloves garlic
5 stalks celery, diced
2 tbsp. extra virgin olive oil
Salt and pepper to taste

Follow these simple steps:

1. Prepare the tofu by taking it out of the package and

blotting with a paper towel until most of the moisture is gone.
2. Bring a skillet to medium heat; crumble the tofu and cook until browned.
3. In a big saucepan, heat the olive oil under medium heat, add celery, and cook for 4 minutes.
4. Add the celery, paprika, cumin, chili powder, cinnamon, and garlic and sauté for 2 minutes.
5. Next, add the mushrooms, zucchini, and bell peppers and cook for approximately 5 minutes.
6. In the big saucepan add cocoa powder, walnuts, tofu, coconut milk, water, tomatoes, tomato paste, and chipotle and simmer for 20-25 minutes or until thick.
7. Dust with some salt and pepper according to preference.

Creamy Avocado Soup

Total Prep & Cooking Time: 46 min.
Yields: 3 Servings
Nutrition Facts: Calories: 226.3 | Carbohydrates: 5.8 g | Proteins: 3.3 g | Fats: 20 g

Ingredients:

1/3 c. cilantro
1/8 t. black pepper
¼ t. salt
1 lime, juiced
1/3 c. coconut milk
½ c. vegetable stock
¼ c. cucumber
2 cloves garlic
2 avocados

Follow these simple steps:

1. In a blender, add avocado, cucumber, lime juice, cilantro, coconut milk, vegetable stock, and garlic.
2. Blend until completely smooth. If you prefer a thinner soup, add additional vegetable stock.
3. Transfer to a big serving bowl and refrigerate for 30 minutes.
4. Dust some salt and pepper to your taste and serve.

Red Onion Soup

Total Prep & Cooking Time: 20 min.
Yields: 2 Servings
Nutrition Facts: Calories: 521 | Carbohydrates: 15.1 g | Proteins: 11.9 g | Fats: 48.4 g

Ingredients:

2 t. pesto
4 tbsp. walnuts
5 tbsp. olive oil
2 tbsp. lemon juice
2 ½ c. vegetable broth
2 cloves garlic, minced
2 red onions
1 t. oregano

Follow these simple steps:

1. Begin by cutting the onion into thin rings and set to the side.
2. In a big pot, add garlic and onions and sauté for 5 minutes.
3. Add in the vegetable broth, oregano, and lemon juice and bring to a simmer for approximately 10 minutes, stirring occasionally.
4. In a skillet, add some olive oil and walnuts; fry for 3 minutes until toasted. Then add to the soup.
5. Finally, add the rest of the seasoning, including the pesto, according to your preference. Serve piping hot.

Thai Pumpkin Soup

Total Prep & Cooking Time: 20 min.
Yields: 4 Servings
Nutrition Facts: Calories: 361 | Carbohydrates: 24.9 g | Proteins: 9.4 g | Fats: 27 g

Ingredients:

1 red chili pepper sliced
13.5 oz. coconut milk
30 oz. pumpkin puree, can
4 c. vegetable broth
2 tbsp. red curry paste

Follow these simple steps:

1. Sit a big saucepan over medium heat; cook the curry paste for about 60 seconds or until the kitchen smells like curry heaven.
2. Pour in the broth, including the pumpkin, stirring to integrate the flavors.
3. Under the same heat setting, wait for the soup to bubble slightly. That's your cue to add the coconut milk. When combined, cook for about 3 minutes.
4. Finally, add to individual bowls and garnish with sliced red chili pepper. Enjoy hot.

Zucchini Basil Soup

Total Prep & Cooking Time: 20 min.
Yields: 4 Servings
Nutrition Facts: Calories: 200 | Carbohydrates: 18 g | Proteins: 3 g | Fats: 14.3 g

Ingredients:

1 c. basil leaves
¾ t. salt
2 c. water
4 cloves garlic
1 ½ pound sliced zucchini
½ t. apple cider vinegar
2 tbsp. olive oil
1 onion, diced

Follow these simple steps:

1. Place a medium-size saucepan over medium-high heat.
2. Sauté the onions and garlic for 2 minutes.
3. Add zucchini and water to the pan and bring to a simmer, cover, and cook for 15 minutes, stirring occasionally.
4. Remove from the heat, and using a hand blender, carefully add in the basil and blend until smooth.
5. Once smooth, add in vinegar and salt and pepper to taste.
6. Finally, add to individual bowls and enjoy.

Chapter 9: Smoothies

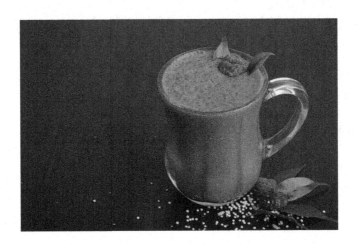

Chocolate Smoothie

Total Prep & Cooking Time: 5 min.
Yields: 2 Servings
Nutrition Facts: Calories: 147 | Carbohydrates: 8.2 g | Proteins: 4 g | Fats: 13.4 g

Ingredients:

¼ c. almond butter
¼ c. cocoa powder, unsweetened
½ c. coconut milk, canned
1 c. almond milk, unsweetened

Follow these simple steps:

1. Before making the smoothie, freeze the almond mı into cubes using an ice cube tray. This would take a few hours, so prepare it ahead.
2. Blend everything using your preferred machine until it reaches your desired thickness.
3. Serve immediately and enjoy!

Chocolate Mint Smoothie

Total Prep & Cooking Time: 5 min.
Yields: 1 Serving
Nutrition Facts: Calories: 401 | Carbohydrates: 6.3 g | Proteins: 5 g | Fats: 40.3 g

Ingredients:

2 tbsp. sweetener of your choice
2 drops mint extract
1 tbsp. cocoa powder
½ avocado, medium
¼ c. coconut milk
1 c. almond milk, unsweetened

Follow these simple steps:
1. In a high-speed blender, add all the ingredients and blend until smooth.
2. Add two to four ice cubes and blend.
3. Serve immediately and enjoy!

Roll Smoothie

Cooking Time: 2 min.

ing

Nutrition Facts: Calories: 507 | Carbohydrates: 17 g | Proteins: 33.3 g | Fats: 34.9 g

Ingredients:

1 t. cinnamon
1 scoop vanilla protein powder
½ c. of the following:
- almond milk, unsweetened
- coconut milk

Sweetener of your choice

Follow these simple steps:
1. In a high-speed blender, add all the ingredients and blend.
2. Add two to four ice cubes and blend until smooth.
3. Serve immediately and enjoy!

Coconut Smoothie

Total Prep & Cooking Time: 2 min.
Yields: 2 Servings
Nutrition Facts: Calories: 584 | Carbohydrates: 22.5 g | Proteins: 8.3 g | Fats: 55.5 g

Ingredients:

1 t. chia seeds
1/8 c. almonds, soaked
1 c. coconut milk
1 avocado

Follow these simple steps:
1. In a high-speed blender, add all the ingredients and blend until smooth.
2. Add your desired number of ice cubes, depending on your favored consistency, of course, and blend again.
3. Serve immediately and enjoy!

Maca Almond Smoothie

Total Prep & Cooking Time: 5 min.
Yields: 2 Servings
Nutrition Facts: Calories: 758 | Carbohydrates: 28.6 g | Proteins: 9.3 g | Fats: 72.3 g

Ingredients:

½ t. vanilla extract
1 scoop maca powder
1 tbsp. almond butter
1 c. almond milk, unsweetened
2 avocados

Follow these simple steps:
1. In a high-speed blender, add all the ingredients and blend until smooth.
2. Serve immediately and enjoy!

Blueberry Smoothie

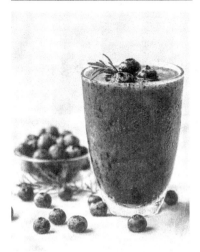

Total Prep & Cooking Time: 5 min.
Yields: 1 Serving
Nutrition Facts: Calories: 401 | Carbohydrates: 6.3 g | Proteins: 5 g | Fats: 40.3 g

Ingredients:

¼ c. pumpkin seeds shelled unsalted
3 c. blueberries, frozen
2 avocados, peeled and halved
1 c. almond milk

Follow these simple steps:
1. In a high-speed blender, add all the ingredients and blend until smooth.
2. Add two to four ice cubes and blend until smooth.
3. Serve immediately and enjoy!

Nutty Protein Shake

Total Prep & Cooking Time: 5 min.
Yields: 1 Serving
Nutrition Facts: Calories: 694 | Carbohydrates: 30.8 g | Proteins: 40.8 g | Fats: 52 g

Ingredients:

¼ avocado
2 tbsp. powdered peanut butter
1 tbsp. of the following:
- Cocoa powder
- Peanut butter

1 scoop protein powder
½ c. almond milk

Follow these simple steps:
1. In a high-speed blender, add all the ingredients and blend until smooth.
2. Add two to four ice cubes and blend again.
3. Serve immediately and enjoy!

Cinnamon Pear Smoothie

Total Prep & Cooking Time: 2 min.
Yields: 1 Serving
Nutrition Facts: Calories: 653 | Carbohydrates: 75.2 g | Proteins: 28.4 g | Fats: 32.2 g

Ingredients:

1 t. cinnamon
1 scoop vanilla protein powder
½ c. of the following:
- Almond milk, unsweetened
- Coconut Milk

2 pears, cores removed
Sweetener of your choice

Follow these simple steps:
1. In a high-speed blender, add all the ingredients and blend.
2. Add two or more ice cubes and blend again.
3. Serve immediately and enjoy!

Vanilla Milkshake

Total Prep & Cooking Time: 5 min.
Yields: 4 Servings
Nutrition Facts: Calories: 125 | Carbohydrates: 6.8 g | Proteins: 1.2 g | Fats: 11.5 g

Ingredients:

2 c. ice cubes
2 t. vanilla extract
6 tbsp. powdered erythritol
1 c. cream of dairy-free
½ c. coconut milk

Follow these simple steps:
1. In a high-speed blender, add all the ingredients and blend.
2. Add ice cubes and blend until smooth.
3. Serve immediately and enjoy!

Raspberry Protein Shake

Total Prep & Cooking Time: 5 min.
Yields: 1 Serving
Nutrition Facts: Calories: 756 | Carbohydrates: 80.1 g | Proteins: 27.6 g | Fats: 40.7 g

Ingredients:

¼ avocado
1 c. raspberries, frozen
1 scoop protein powder
½ c. almond milk
Ice cubes

Follow these simple steps:
1. In a high-speed blender add all the ingredients and blend until lumps of fruit disappear.
2. Add two to four ice cubes and blend to your desired consistency.
3. Serve immediately and enjoy!

Raspberry Almond Smoothie

Total Prep & Cooking Time: 5 min.
Yields: 1 Serving
Nutrition Facts: Calories: 449 | Carbohydrates: 26 g | Proteins: 14 g | Fats: 35 g

Ingredients:

10 Almonds, finely chopped
3 tbsp. almond butter
1 c. almond milk
1 c. Raspberries, frozen

Follow these simple steps:
1. In a high-speed blender, add all the ingredients and blend until smooth.
2. Serve immediately and enjoy!

Chapter 10: Desserts

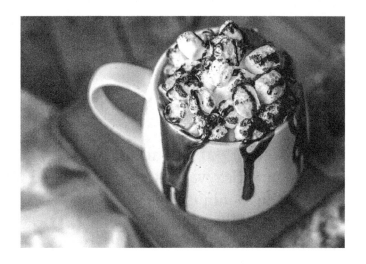

Keto Chocolate Brownies

Total Prep & Cooking Time: 30 min.
Yields: 16 Servings
Nutrition Facts: Calories: 131 | Carbohydrates: 12.3 g | Proteins: 1.8 g | Fats: 8.8 g

Ingredients:

¼ t. of the following:
- salt
- baking soda

½ c. of the following:
- sweetener of your choice
- coconut flour
- vegetable oil
- water

¼ c. of the following:
- cocoa powder
- almond milk yogurt

1 tbsp. ground flax
1 t. vanilla extract

Follow these simple steps:

1. Bring the oven to 350 heat setting.
2. Mix the ground flax, vanilla, yogurt, oil, and water; set to the side for 10 minutes.
3. Line an oven-safe 8x8 baking dish with parchment paper.
4. After 10 minutes have passed, add coconut flour, cocoa powder, sweetener, baking soda, and salt.
5. Bake for 15 minutes; make sure that you placed it in the center. When they come out, they will look underdone.
6. Place in the refrigerator and let them firm up overnight.

Chocolate Fat Bomb

Total Prep & Cooking Time: 5 min.
Yields: 14 Servings
Nutrition Facts: Calories: 84 | Carbohydrates: 2.6 g | Proteins: 2 g | Fats: 8.2 g

Ingredients:

1 tbsp. liquid sweetener of your choice.
¼ c. of the following:
- coconut oil, melted
- cocoa powder

½ c. almond butter

Follow these simple steps:

1. Mix the ingredients in a medium bowl until smooth. Pour into the candy molds or ice cube trays.
2. Put in the freezer to set.
3. Store in freezer.

Vanilla Cheesecake

Total Prep & Cooking Time: 3 hr. 20 min.
Yields: 10 Servings
Nutrition Facts: Calories: 300 | Carbohydrates: 7.7 g | Proteins: 7.1 g | Fats: 28.3 g

Ingredients:

1 tbsp. vanilla extract,
2 ½ tbsp. lemon juice
½ c. coconut oil
1/8 t. stevia powder
6 tbsp. coconut milk
1 ½ c. blanched almonds soaked

Crust:
2 tbsp. coconut oil
1 ½ c. almonds

Follow these simple steps:

For the Crust:

1. In a food processor, add the almonds and coconut oil and pulse until crumbles start to form.
2. Line a 7-inch springform pan with parchment paper and firmly press the crust into the bottom.

For the Sauce:

3. Bring a saucepan of water to a boil and soak the almonds for 2 hours. Drain and shake to dry.

4. Next, add the almonds to the food processor and blend until completely smooth.
5. Add vanilla, lemon, coconut oil, stevia, and coconut milk and blend until smooth.
6. Pour over the crust and freeze overnight or for a minimum of 3 hours.
7. Serve and enjoy.

Chocolate Mousse

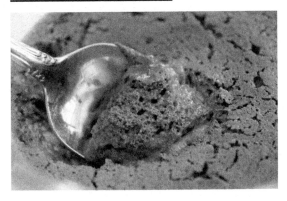

Total Prep & Cooking Time: 5 min.
Yields: 2 Servings
Nutrition Facts: Calories: 420| Carbohydrates: 13.5 g | Proteins: 6.2 g | Fats: 42.9 g

Ingredients:

6 drops liquid stevia extract
½ t. cinnamon
3 tbsp. cocoa powder, unsweetened
1 c. coconut milk

Follow these simple steps:

1. On the day before, place the coconut milk into the refrigerator overnight.
2. Remove the coconut milk from the refrigerator; it should be very thick.
3. Whisk in cocoa powder with an electric mixer.
4. Add stevia and cinnamon and whip until combined.
5. Place in individual bowls and serve and enjoy.

Avocado Chocolate Mousse

Total Prep & Cooking Time: 3 hr. 20 min.
Yields: 4 Servings
Nutrition Facts: Calories: 343 | Carbohydrates: 12 g | Proteins: 3.3 g | Fats: 33.9 g

Ingredients:

2 pinches sea salt
4 tbsp. sweetener of your choice
1 c. almond milk, unsweetened
2 avocados, peeled and pitted

Follow these simple steps:

1. Blend everything using a machine of your choice, as long as the consistency becomes smooth for a mousse. If too thick, add some more coconut milk, ¼ teaspoon at a time.
2. Serve and enjoy.

Coconut Fat Bombs

Total Prep & Cooking Time: 1 hr. 5 min.
Yields: 4 Servings
Nutrition Facts: Calories: 89.1 | Carbohydrates: 0.87 g | Proteins: 0.33 g | Fats: 9.7 g

Ingredients:

20 drops liquid stevia
1 c. coconut flakes, unsweetened
¾ c. coconut oil
1 can coconut milk

Follow these simple steps:

1. In a big microwave-safe mixing bowl, add coconut oil and warm on low power for 20 seconds to melt.
2. Whisk in coconut milk and stevia into the oil.
3. Add coconut flakes; combine well.
4. Pour into candy molds or ice cube trays and freeze for 1 hour.
5. Serve and enjoy.

Coconut Cupcakes

Total Prep & Cooking Time: 1 hr. 5 min.
Yields: 18 Servings
Nutrition Facts: Calories: 202 | Carbohydrates: 15.6 g | Proteins: 3.3 g | Fats: 15.8 g

Ingredients:

1 tbsp. vanilla
1 t. baking soda
1 c. erythritol
4 t. baking powder
1 ¼ c. coconut milk
¾ c. coconut flour
14 tbsp. arrowroot powder
2 c. almond meal
½ c. coconut oil

Whipped Cream:

1 t. vanilla
¼ c. erythritol
2 13.5 oz. cans full-fat coconut milk, refrigerated overnight

Follow these simple steps:

1. Prepare a muffin tin with muffin liners and bring the oven to 350 heat setting.
2. In a big mixing bowl, add all the ingredients and beat on medium-high speed until it turns to a batter-like

consistency. If too dry, add ¼ teaspoon of water at a time.
3. Fill the cupcake cups with the batter, three-quarters full.
4. Bake for 20 minutes or until the cupcakes are firm.
5. Place in the refrigerator to cool.
6. While cupcakes are cooling, make the whipped cream.
7. Remove the coconut milk from the fridge and pour the clear coconut water from the milk.
8. In a big mixing bowl, add the vanilla and erythritol; beat until fluffy.
9. Ice the cupcakes and serve.
10. Serve and enjoy.

Pumpkin Truffles

Total Prep & Cooking Time: 15 min.
Yields: 12 Servings
Nutrition Facts: Calories: 66 | Carbohydrates: 10 g | Proteins: 1 g | Fats: 2 g

Ingredients:

1 t. cinnamon
2 tbsp. coconut sugar
3 tbsp. coconut flour
½ c. almond flour
1 t. pumpkin pie spice
¼ t. salt
½ t. vanilla extract
¼ c. maple syrup

1 c. pumpkin puree

Follow these simple steps:

1. Bring a saucepan to medium heat and add pumpkin puree, syrup, salt, and pumpkin pie spice, stirring constantly until thickened about 5 minutes.
2. Once thick, add in vanilla and continue to stir for an additional minute.
3. Remove from the heat and allow to cool.
4. Once cool, mix in the coconut and almond flour. Then put in the refrigerator to chill for 10 minutes.
5. Remove from the fridge and mix again. If the dough is too sticky, add in 1 tablespoon of almond flour until you can form a ball with the dough.
6. Form 12 balls using your hands with the dough.
7. In a little bowl, combine coconut sugar and cinnamon.
8. Roll each ball into the cinnamon-sugar mixture.
9. Serve and enjoy.

<u>Raspberry Truffles</u>

Total Prep & Cooking Time: 15 min.
Yields: 36 Servings
Nutrition Facts: Calories: 39 | Carbohydrates: 3.8 g | Proteins: 0.6 g | Fats: 2.6 g

Ingredients:

2 tbsp. cocoa powder, unsweetened

6 oz. of the following:
- fresh raspberries, dry
- chocolate, bittersweet, finely chopped
- coconut milk, full-fat

Follow these simple steps:

1. Prepare a cookie sheet with parchment paper and set to the side.
2. Warm a saucepan over medium heat, and add coconut milk.
3. Remove from the heat and add the chocolate with a rubber spatula, stirring to melt the chocolate
4. Once smooth, add the raspberries, 5-8 at a time. Stir to coat.
5. Using two forks, remove the raspberries from the chocolate sauce, allowing the excess sauce to drop back into the pan. Repeat this step until you have coated all raspberries.
6. Place the raspberries in the refrigerator for 1 hour or until firm.
7. In a shallow bowl with a lid, add the cocoa powder.
8. Once truffles are firm, place 5 to 8 truffles in the bowl and shake to coat with cocoa powder.
9. Return to the refrigerator until ready to serve.

Strawberry Ice Cream

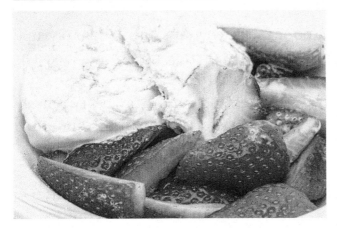

Total Prep & Cooking Time: 7 hr. 60 min.
Yields: 8 Servings
Nutrition Facts: Calories: 273 | Carbohydrates: 23.9 g | Proteins: 1.4 g | Fats: 19.4 g

Ingredients:

½ t. salt
1 tbsp. strawberry extract
1 c. strawberry puree
¼ c. maple syrup
½ c. sweetener of your choice
14 oz. coconut milk
14 oz. coconut cream

You will need an ice cream maker for this recipe.

Follow these simple steps:

1. Place your ice cream bowl in the freezer one day before.
2. In a saucepan, pour in the coconut milk, sugar, syrup, and coconut cream, gently stirring until it reaches a simmer. Then remove from the heat.
3. Add in salt, strawberry extract, and strawberry puree then blend with an immersion blender until smooth.
4. Transfer the mixture into a container with a lid and place in the freezer to chill for 30 minutes.
5. Following the directions on your ice cream maker, churn the mixture for about 20-40 minutes until a soft-serve consistency is reached.
6. Transfer to a loaf pan and place in the freezer for approximately 6 hours.
7. Scoop and serve.

Pistachio Gelato

Total Prep & Cooking Time: 7 hr. 60 min.
Yields: 4 Servings
Nutrition Facts: Calories: 345 | Carbohydrates: 38.8 g | Proteins: 6.5 g | Fats: 19.8 g

Ingredients:

½ t. almond extract
1 c. of the following:
- Medjool dates
- pistachios, unsalted, shells removed

1 big avocado
2 ½ c. cashew milk

Follow these simple steps:

1. In a blender, add almond extract, dates, pistachios, avocado, and milk and blend until smooth.
2. Once smooth, pour into a loaf pan, topping with chopped pistachios and freeze for 8 hours or overnight.
3. Remove from the freezer and allow to fall for 15 minutes before serving.
4. Scoop and serve.

Chocolate Chip Ice Cream

Total Prep & Cooking Time: 7 hr. 60 min.
Yields: 8 Servings
Nutrition Facts: Calories: 429 | Carbohydrates: 48.2 g | Proteins: 3.3 g | Fats: 26.2 g

Ingredients:

½ t. salt
1 c. chocolate chips
¼ c. maple syrup
½ c. sweetener of your choice
14 oz. of the following:
- Coconut milk
- Coconut cream

You will need an ice cream maker for this recipe.

Follow these simple steps:

1. Place your ice cream bowl in the freezer on the day before.
2. In a saucepan, add coconut milk, sugar, syrup, and coconut cream, gently stirring until it reaches a simmer. Then remove from heat.
3. Add in salt and blend with an immersion blender until smooth.
4. Transfer mixture into a container with a lid and place in the freezer to chill for 15 minutes.

5. Remove from the freezer and fold in the chocolate chips. Place back in the freezer for an additional 15 minutes
6. Following the directions on your ice cream maker, churn the mixture for about 20-40 minutes until a soft-serve consistency is reached.
7. Transfer to a loaf pan and place in the freezer for approximately 6 hours.
8. Scoop and serve.

Cinnamon Vanilla Bites

Total Prep & Cooking Time: 60 min.
Yields: 15 Servings
Nutrition Facts: Calories: 194 | Carbohydrates: 8.9 g | Proteins: 11.9 g | Fats: 14.4 g

Ingredients:

2 tbsp. water
1 t. vanilla extract
1 tbsp. cinnamon
¼ c. of the following:
- vanilla vegan protein powder
- maple syrup

½ c. of the following:
- almonds, unsalted
- almond butter

¾ c hemp hearts

For coating:
1 t cinnamon + 1 tbsp. vanilla protein powder

Follow these simple steps:

1. In a food processor, add vanilla, cinnamon, protein powder, syrup, almonds, almond butter, and hemp hearts and blend until combined.
2. Add water, ½ tablespoon at a time, until the mixture begins to stick together and form a ball.
3. Using your hands, form 1 ½ inch balls.

4. In a shallow bowl with a lid, combine 1 teaspoon cinnamon and 2 tablespoons of protein powder.
5. Add a few balls at a time to the bowl and coat with the powder mixture.
6. Store in refrigerator and serve cool.

Berry Bites

Total Prep & Cooking Time: 60 min.
Yields: 13 Servings
Nutrition Facts: Calories: 75 | Carbohydrates: 2.8 g | Proteins: 0.8 g | Fats: 7.2 g

Ingredients:

Dash Himalayan pink salt
1/16 t. stevia
½ t. vanilla
½ c. blackberries
2/3 c. coconut butter

Follow these simple steps:

1. In a food processor, add coconut butter, blackberries, vanilla, stevia, and salt; blend until well combined.
2. Using your hands, form them into 1 ½-inch balls, and place them on parchment a paper on a flat dish.
3. Place the dish in the freezer for 15 minutes to set.
4. Store in refrigerator and serve cool.

Coconut Chocolate Balls

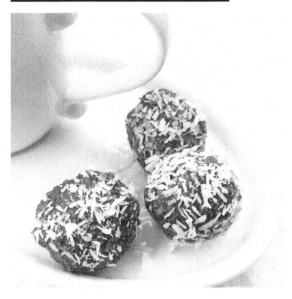

Total Prep & Cooking Time: 20 min.
Yields: 22 Servings
Nutrition Facts: Calories: 179 | Carbohydrates: 18.6 g | Proteins: 6 g | Fats: 10.2 g

Ingredients:

¼ c. of the following:
- coconut, unsweetened, finely shredded
- coconut oil, melted

16 oz. Medjool dates
1 1/3 c. hemp hearts
¼ t. sea salt, ground
2 tbsp. ground flaxseed
½ c. cocoa, unsweetened
¾ c. almonds, sliced

Follow these simple steps:

1. In a food processor, finely chop the almonds for 30 seconds.
2. Next, add in the hemp hearts, sea salt, flaxseed, and cocoa and blend for another 30 seconds.
3. Add in the coconut oil and dates; blend it for 2 minutes or until well-blended. If the mixture is not sticking together, add ¼ t. of coconut oil until sticky.
4. Using your hands, form them into 1 ½-inch balls.
5. Place on a paper-lined dish and store into the freezer for 15 minutes to set.
6. In a shallow bowl, place finely shredded coconut. Roll each ball into the coconut, pressing gently but firmly.
7. Store in the refrigerator and serve cool.

Espresso Cups

Total Prep & Cooking Time: 20 min.
Yields: 22 Servings
Nutrition Facts: Calories: 77 | Carbohydrates: 1 g | Proteins: 1 g | Fats: 8 g

Ingredients:

15 drops vanilla stevia
1 ½ tbsp. instant espresso powder
1 tbsp. coconut milk
2 tbsp. cocoa powder
1/3 c. of the following:
- coconut oil
- almond butter

Follow these simple steps:

1. In a saucepan over medium-low heat, melt the almond butter, coconut oil, coconut powder, coconut milk, espresso powder, and stevia. Stir frequently not to scorch.
2. Pour into the candy molds or ice cube trays and freeze for 30 minutes.
3. Store in the refrigerator and serve cool.

Conclusion

I hope you found your copy of *Keto-Vegan Cookbook for Beginners* helpful. I hope you found some sections informative and were provided lots of great new tools to help you live your keto-vegan lifestyle. I say "lifestyle" because the word diet is not really appropriate. If you want to find success in healthy living, it has to be a lifestyle choice, not simply a diet that will end at some given date in the future. Living on the keto-vegan lifestyle offers so many different physical and health benefits, along with the opportunity to expand your taste buds to different spices and cuisines you may have never considered.

The next step is to prepare that shopping list and head to the market. Be sure to pay attention to what might be seasonally prepared and when those ingredients are the freshest. The fresher the ingredients are, the better the dish. Always look for organic or naturally sourced produce to make sure you are getting top-quality freshness.

Before you know it, you will be the envy of the neighborhood with your delicious healthy meals and amazing desserts. Taking steps to better your health is a hard choice to make. Congratulations, you have done the hard part and have taken that first step to a better life. Using this book, you will not only have a variety of dishes to satisfy your taste buds, but you might also surprise your carnivore friends.

Index for the Recipes

Chapter 4: Breakfast Choices

Strawberry Porridge
Gingerbread Porridge
Overnight Strawberry Cheesecake Porridge
Blueberry Quinoa Porridge
Blueberry Chia Pudding
Almond Flour Muffins
Bulletproof Tea
Bulletproof Coffee
Coconut Pancakes
Flaxseed Pancakes
Berry and Nut Cereal
Peanut Butter Fudgy Brownies
Vanilla Golden Turmeric Cereal
Fudge Oatmeal
Raspberry Almond Smoothie
Vanilla Overnight Oats
Cinnamon Overnight Oats
Pumpkin Spice Overnight Oats
Smoothie Bowl
Eggy Surprise Scramble
Bagels
Cinnamon Roll Muffins

Chapter 5: Lunch & Dinner Favorites

Mushroom Steak
Spicy Grilled Tofu Steak
Piquillo Salsa Verde Steak
Butternut Squash Steak
Cauliflower Steak Kicking Corn
Pistachio Watermelon Steak
BBQ Ribs
Spicy Veggie Steaks With veggies
Tofu Seitan
Stuffed Zucchini
Roasted Butternut Squash With Chimichurri
Eggplant Pizza
Green Avocado Carbonara
Curried Tofu
Sesame Tofu and Eggplant
Tempeh Coconut Curry
Tempeh Tikka Masala
Caprice Casserole
Cheesy Brussel Sprout Bake
Tofu Noodle Bowl
Cashew Siam Salad
Cucumber Edamame Salad
Caesar Vegan Salad
Mushroom Lettuce Wraps

Chapter 6: Side Dishes & Snacks

Mixed Seed Crackers
Crispy Squash Chips
Paprika Nuts
Basil Zoodles and Olives

Roasted Beetroot Noodles
Turnip Fries
Lime and Chili Carrots Noodles
Pesto Zucchini Noodles
Cabbage Slaw
Zucchini Chips
Peanut Tofu Wrap
Cinnamon Granola
Chocolate Granola
Radish Chips
Asparagus Fries

Chapter 7: Sauces & Dips

Keto-Vegan Ketchup
Avocado Hummus
Guacamole
Keto-Vegan Mayo
Peanut Sauce
Pistachio Dip
Smokey Tomato Jam
Tasty Ranch Dressing/Dip

Chapter 8: Soups

Goulash Soup
Celery Dill Soup
Broccoli Fennel Soup
Broccoli and Cauliflower Soup
Keto-Vegan Chili
Creamy Avocado Soup

Red Onion Soup
Thai Pumpkin Soup
Zucchini Basil Soup

Chapter 9: Smoothies

Chocolate Smoothie
Chocolate Mint Smoothie
Cinnamon Roll Smoothie
Coconut Smoothie
Maca Almond Smoothie
Blueberry Smoothie
Nutty Protein Shake
Cinnamon Pear Smoothie
Vanilla Milkshake
Raspberry Protein Shake
Raspberry Almond Smoothie

Chapter 10 Deserts

Keto Chocolate Brownies
Chocolate Fat Bomb
Vanilla Cheesecake
Chocolate Mousse
Avocado Chocolate Mousse
Coconut Fat Bombs
Coconut Cupcakes
Pumpkin Truffles
Raspberry Truffles
Strawberry Ice Cream
Pistachio Gelato

Chocolate Chip Ice Cream
Cinnamon Vanilla Bites
Berry Bites
Coconut Chocolate Balls
Espresso Cups

Keto for Women Over 50

The Ultimate Guide for Senior Women to Ketogenic Diet and a Healthy Weight Loss, Including Mouthwatering Recipes to Reset Your Metabolism and Boost your Energy

Thomas Slow

Introduction

Congratulations on purchasing *Keto For Women Over 50,* and thank you for doing so.

This book is for women over 50 looking to lose weight and increase energy levels through the ketogenic (keto) diet. Naysayers will say the keto diet is a fad, but some form of this diet has been used for various health purposes, including weight loss, since 1825. Over the last 200 years, the diet has been changed and adjusted to incorporate the newest scientific information into the diet. As a result, the keto diet takes an age-old concept of limiting carbohydrates with the current knowledge of how fats work in the human body and now the diet is better than ever. The weight loss, when adapting the keto diet, is almost immediate. This book provides a basic framework for losing weight and improving your health by adopting a low-carbohydrate, high-fat diet. Your questions will be answered. By now, you've probably realized that it is not as easy to lose weight as it was when you were younger. That is probably the result of a lot of things; a slowing metabolism and decreased mobility are the obvious reasons you may be gaining weight, but the food you eat may be a culprit as well. Reading this book, you will be able to completely restructure your life and diet to follow ketogenic principles. The ketogenic diet is designed to help you lose weight with an increased energy level. This book outlines the basics and has the information to get you started. As a bonus, you will receive over 20 recipes that follow the keto diet principles. These recipes give you an opportunity to find new and creative ways to prepare food when you are starting out and may not be familiar with all the foods on the plan. There is also a food list inside that you can use to plan meals and purchase groceries for your new lighter, healthier lifestyle.

There happens to be a lot of books out there on this subject. Thank you for purchasing this one! I made sure it is jam packed with helpful information to get you where you want to be. Enjoy!

Chapter 1: Keto – An Overview

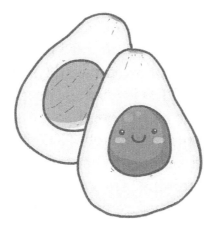

What is the Keto Diet?

Before you start the ketogenic diet, you will want to know what it is. The diet, at its most basic, is the replacement of carbohydrates with fats. This makes the keto diet not only a low carb diet but a very low carb diet. The food consumed on the keto diet will be high in fat with the reduction of carbs. When you limit the number of carbohydrates in your body, you will get your energy from stored fat. This is called ketosis. When your body is in ketosis, it is in a metabolic state that causes it to burn fat for energy instead of carbohydrates. This is the state we strive to reach on the diet; energy from fat.

There are four types of keto diets:

1. The standard ketogenic diet (SKD) is the basic ketogenic diet. This diet allows for 75% of the calories consumed to be from fat, 20% of the calories from protein, and 5% carbohydrates.
2. The cyclical ketogenic diet (CKD) is designed so that the dieter follows the Standard Ketogenic Diet for 5 days each week, followed by 2 days of high carbohydrates. CKD is used for people attempting to increase muscle and strength.
3. The targeted ketogenic diet (TKD) is used by people who need extra energy to get through strenuous workouts or training. The carbohydrates can be consumed either before or after a workout to provide extra energy for the short term.
4. On the high protein ketogenic diet (HPKD) is used for people who do not want to lose muscle mass like bodybuilders and older people. The percentage of protein in the diet can go up to 35% with fat decreasing as low as 60%, with the carbohydrates remaining at 5%.

The ketogenic diet is based on science. When the body does not have carbohydrates to use as energy, fat is used instead. This process is called ketogenesis, and the body generates. During this process, ketones are generated by the liver. The average person can safely get up to 70% of its energy from ketones. It takes about three weeks for the body to transform itself from using carbohydrates for energy to efficiently using ketones for energy.

What is Ketosis?

Ketosis is a metabolic state where the body is efficiently using fat for energy. In a regular diet, carbohydrates produce glucose, which is used to provide energy. Glucose is stored in the body in fat cells that travel via the bloodstream. People gain weight when there is more fat stored than being used as energy.

Glucose is formed through the consumption of sugar and starch. Namely carbohydrates. The sugars may be in the form of natural sugars from fruit or milk, or they may be formed from processed sugar. Starches like pasta, rice or starchy vegetables like potatoes and corn, form glucose as well. The body breaks down the sugars from these foods into glucose. Glucose and insulin combined to help to carry glucose into the bloodstream so the body can use glucose as energy. The glucose that is not used is stored in the liver and muscles.

In order for the body to supply ketones for use as fuel, the body must use up all the reserves of glucose. In order to do this, there must be a condition of the body of starvation low carbohydrates, passing, or strenuous exercise. A very low carb diet, the production of ketones what her to feel the body and brain.

Ketones are produced from the liver when there is not enough glucose in the body to provide energy. When insulin levels are low, and there is not enough glucose or sugar in the bloodstream, fat is released from fat cells and travels in the blood to the liver. The liver processes the fat into ketones. Ketones are released into the bloodstream to provide fuel for the body and increase the body's metabolism. Ketones are formed under conditions of starvation, fasting, or a diet low in carbohydrates. As ketones are formed, they use the fatty acids, triglycerides, to produce high levels of energy to the muscles, heart, and brain.

Ketones are naturally produced in the body under normal dieting circumstances. The heart and kidney prefer the energy produced from ketones. This is because ketones utilize slow-release energy that is sustained over a long period of time. Glucose energy, which tends to be quick spurts of energy, is less efficient. When ketones are used to fuel the brain, cognitive function can improve and may have a positive impact on brain issues like Parkinson's and dementia. Studies are being done to determine the effectiveness of ketones and ketosis on improving brain function.

How is Insulin Affected by the Keto Diet?

In order to achieve ketosis, insulin production must be minimized. Insulin inhibits the production of ketones. In a normal body, one that doesn't require the introduction of insulin from outside the body, insulin is released from the pancreas, the response to certain foods being consumed. In order to reduce the need for insulin to be released, the diet must be changed so that there are only a few carbs, as few as possible. At the same time, there should only as much protein in the body as it needs in a daily diet.

When a person consumes carbohydrates, the glucose in the carbohydrates is released into the bloodstream. This causes the blood sugar levels to rise in the pancreas to produce insulin into the bloodstream so that the glucose is able to travel through the body and distribute the energy. Leftover glucose that has not been turned into energy becomes stored in fat cells for another time. The stored fat is available then converted to energy when it is called for. For people with type 1 diabetes, the pancreas doesn't make enough insulin to take care of the glucose and blood sugar levels remain high, presenting a dangerous health situation.

Insulin may also be released from the pancreas if there is excess protein in the blood. For this reason, the keto diet stresses the consumption of moderate amounts of protein, and it is important to eat the right combination of protein. The keto diet allows for the consumption of high fat and low protein to provide the optimal combination to enter ketosis. Protein is important for the development of muscle and tissue. Too much protein produces insulin, which inhibits the production of ketones. It is important to provide your body with the correct amount of protein a low amount of carbohydrates. Reducing the grams of carbohydrates eaten minimizes the need for sudden influxes of insulin into the system. In fact, can be reduced over a sustained time period without long-term adverse effects on the body and its health.

Positive Effects of the Keto Diet

The keto diet may have several positive effects on the body. One of the most prominent positive aspects of the keto diet is the ease of sticking to the diet. Successful weight loss plans must be easy to follow for most people to be successful. A low-carb diet may be easy to follow because the keto diet can greatly reduce appetite. If you don't feel hungry, you're more likely to stay on the diet plan. When a person consumes carbohydrates, there is a burst of energy and a feeling of fullness. Unfortunately, these sensations are short-lived because the glucose used to generate energy burns away quickly. This leads to hunger within a short time span. While on keto, the fats will keep you feeling full for a longer period of time. Additionally, as long as you are snacking on items within the plan, there is a lot of room for high-fat items in the diet.

Another good thing about the keto diet, especially in the beginning, you will lose weight. By staying on the plan and following the tenets, you're likely to lose up to twice as much weight at the beginning of a diet as you will with low-fat, low-calorie diets. This is especially true during the first two or three weeks on the diet as the body sheds excess water.

The keto diet reduces the amount of fat stored in the body. The fat loss is made up of visceral fat. Visceral fat is fat that accumulates in the abdomen and tends to attach itself to organs. The keto diet may reduce the fat, which is known to be the most harmful and may reduce the risk of heart disease and type 2 diabetes. These issues are often seen in people who are obese or simply overweight. The visceral fat loss reduces the fat in the most harmful areas of the body and improves overall health in many individuals.

Finally, diets focusing on low carbohydrate consumption will almost always reduce blood sugar levels and improve blood pressure. Carbohydrates increase blood sugar levels. In response to the high blood sugar levels, insulin is produced to regulate blood sugar levels into a normal range. By minimizing the carbohydrates introduced into the bloodstream, your body is not exposed to the spikes of sugar in the bloodstream and effectively reduces the amount of insulin needed to combat the sugar spikes. This will also be instrumental in avoiding the energy lows that are experienced when the carbohydrate energy is burned off. Blood pressure may be positively affected by the keto diet as well. It is important to consume fats that are high in good cholesterol as opposed to bad cholesterol. Good cholesterol is usually present in fats found in plant products like avocados. It has also been found that reducing the consumption of carbohydrates also raises the amount of good cholesterol, HDL, and lowers the amount of bad cholesterol, LDL, in your body.

__Negative Effects of Keto__

Along with the dramatic change in diet, there may be some negative experiences on the ketogenic diet. One of the more common issues is keto flu. This is a general feeling of fatigue that may accompany entering ketosis. This feeling of tiredness may be accompanied by nausea and upset stomach. It is a common reaction to the body as it adapts to reduced carbohydrates and the switch to getting energy from ketones instead of glucose.

Besides the keto flu, there may also be keto diarrhea. This is likely caused by the gallbladder producing more bile to deal with increased fat consumption. Until the body adjusts to the increased amounts of fat and enters ketosis, diarrhea may be a side effect. Diarrhea may also result from a reduction in the amount of fiber ingested because of a decrease in carbohydrate consumption. The fiber from carbs must be replaced with fiber from low-carb vegetables. This will help mitigate issues with diarrhea resulting from the lack of carbohydrates and, therefore fiber in the diet.

One way to reduce gastrointestinal issues associated with the keto diet is to make sure you drink plenty of water. It is important to stay hydrated and flush out your system. Drinking lots of water helps to remove toxins from the body before they have time to linger in organs and tissues.

The keto diet will precipitate weight loss. Unfortunately, this weight loss may include the reduction of muscle mass as well as fat. This is not ideal, especially for women over 50 in whom muscle mass begins to atrophy naturally. Additionally, reduced muscle mass may change your metabolism because you burn more calories with muscle than fat. This loss of muscle is more likely to happen if you are consuming more fat than protein. The type of fat consumed will be important to retain muscle mass as you lose weight. This will be addressed in a later section of this book.

Keto Mistakes

The most common mistakes revolve around food choices. It is important to maintain correct ratios of fats to proteins. The diet program is subject to fail, and poor health may result in failing to maintain the proper amount of fat. The ketogenic diet is based on using fat to burn as fuel in the body. As a result, the body needs fat to burn. Of course, these need to be good fats that promote increases in HDL cholesterol. This will provide good fuel for the body.

It is important to eat the right fats. Margarine, vegetable oil, canola oil, trans fats, and other light non-viscous plant oils and unhealthy fats should be eliminated from the diet. The fat consumed should be high quality like butter from grass-fed animals, olive oil, monounsaturated oils such as from avocados and coconuts. These are oils and fats are the best options for food and keto. The quality of the fat is important so that it is easily processed and converted to fuel.

Be sure to drink adequate amounts of water when you're on the keto diet. Water will help prevent some of the adverse side effects of the keto diet. It can help with constipation and also help dilute ketones, and acids subject accumulate in the bloodstream. Water is an instrumental factor in avoiding additional weight gain from retention and bloating. You will feel better drinking plenty of water.

Failing to drink adequate amounts of water is a common and unhealthy mistake made by ketogenic dieters. Especially at the beginning of the diet, urination will be frequent. The water needs to be replaced, and you may need to replace electrolytes as well. Make sure to feed your body appropriate nutrients.

When you embark on the keto diet, you may find that you eliminate many processed foods from your diet. These foods use salt as a preservative. Because of this, you will need to replace the salt in your system that you will lose as you drink more water and urinate more frequently. This will help you avoid keto flu or reduce the symptoms of the keto flu.

One of the main mistakes people make on the keto diet is eating too many calories. There is a myth that you can eat whatever you like on the keto diet as long as it is low or no carb and/or high in fat. General life principles are still in effect. If you consume more calories than you burn, you'll gain weight. It is important to maintain vigilance in the number of calories consumed and be sure to eat quality foods containing whole grains and fiber. Though there is room in the diet for keto-friendly snacks, try to avoid processed snacks, which may have more carbohydrates than expected. It is important to review all processed food labels to know the nutritional value of the food you consume.

Chapter 2: Keto for Women Over 50

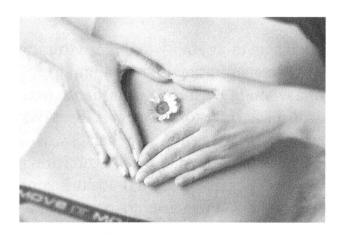

Because of the changes occurring in the bodies of women over 50, it is imperative to look at how the needs of these women are different than younger women and men. During menopause, hormones shift in women, and these changes make it necessary to make some adjustments to their lifestyle in general, and diet in particular.

General Nutritional Needs for Women Over 50

As a woman enters her fifties, it becomes necessary to make modifications to the diet to be healthy. This is because of changes in hormones and metabolism. There is a decrease in muscle mass. To offset this change, there is a need to increase the amount of protein in the diet. At the same time, bone density decreases, making it necessary to increase the amount of vitamin D and calcium consumed in order to maintain adequate bone density as the body ages. All this, combined with a reduction in the number of calories needed to fuel the body, makes it necessary to modify diet as a woman enters postmenopausal years. These natural changes to the body make changes to the diet necessary as a woman ages.

Also, as women age, their ability to discern thirstiness may diminish. Water consumption is still an important factor in the health of a woman. Because it is harder to determine thirst as you surpass your 50th year, it is essential that you consume 8 to 9 8 oz glasses of water each day. Drink more in the winter in hot weather and when exercising. While you are drinking more water, it may serve to curb your appetite. This is good because you will need to lower your caloric intake from what you may be accustomed to. this happens when you are finding new aches and pains and slowing down your exercise regime. Exercise may be less intense as you make modifications to coincide with your age and decreases in mobility. This is because you are not as flexible and may be experiencing inflammation in your joints. While these are all relatively normal signs of aging, the decrease in physical activity may cause additional problems in the form of weight gain.

This may be a good time to eliminate processed foods and sugar from your diet. Dietary fiber is the key to avoiding constipation. Studies show that women over 50 may be up to seven times more likely to suffer from constipation than men of a similar age. Failure to consume enough dietary fiber can result in small, hard stool. It is beneficial to consume dietary fiber, which is found in whole grains, and food is made from whole grains, as well as fruits and vegetables. The foods move through intestines easily and make solid stool that moves through the intestines quickly and efficiently. The dietary fiber in these foods may help in lowering bad cholesterol (LDL) levels in adults. This may have a positive effect on heart health as well. Since estrogen levels in women are also decreasing, the female body begins to lose the positive effect estrogen has on the heart and blood vessels. This is another impact of menopause. Consuming adequate amounts of dietary fiber may help to improve heart health.

Gentler Approach to Keto for Women Over 50

Women over 50 may want to modify their keto approach by increasing the daily carbohydrates to 100 to 150 g each day. They may also want to increase the protein from 25% to 30% of the diet. The remaining amount of food will be fat. The increased carbohydrates provide less distress to hormones and metabolism and put less stress on the body while adjusting to a diet low in carbohydrates. The increase in protein is to offset the body's tendency to lose muscle mass as women age. Additionally, the carbs will provide energy to exercise. The metabolism of women typically slow as women age. The increase in carbs and protein may allow women over 50 to forgo the sluggish feelings and allow enough energy to exercise while on the diet. This will improve overall health.

Carbohydrates in your diet should come from whole grains or high-quality carbs like pumpkins, carrots, spaghetti squash, and small quantities of butternut squash. Foods that grow below the ground have higher carbohydrate content. If you feel like you need to sneak them into your diet, it should be small amounts per serving. They add variety and flavor to your diet, but they must be used in moderation. Even with a few extra carbs in your diet, you should be able to enter ketosis. The same is true for protein. The body may not enter ketosis as quickly, but the effects of the changes will not be as jarring to your body and the internal system of operation.

The keto diet stresses the importance of high fiber low carb food. Be sure to include leafy greens and healthy oils in the diet. The leafy greens will help avoid gastrointestinal issues during keto. They contain the fiber lost with the reduction of carbohydrates. Many vegetables contain carbohydrates, so be aware of the amount you are eating and stay within your macros. Some of the vegetables have fiber and no carbohydrates, but others, like cauliflower and jicama, have carbs. You must remember to count them in your daily totals. Green leafy vegetables have protein that must be added as well. Overall, it is best to get your fiber from vegetables to keep you energized and lessen the effects of keto flu and keto diarrhea, as well as constipation.

Tracking and Macros

Macronutrients are found in every food. They are the nutrients that fuel the body. Carbohydrates, proteins, and fats are included in the calories consumed and should be tracked while on the keto diet. The information needed is on the nutritional value label found on foods. Accurately measure individual portions to be sure to have accurate nutritional information. These nutrients being tracked are typically called "macros" which is a shortened version of the word macronutrient. This book specifies the macros that you need to know for a ketogenic diet plan. By making adjustments to the SKD and HPKD, a gentler keto plan may be created in order to fit the needs of women over 50.

First, we will look at the carbohydrates. You will be counting net carbs. Grams of net carbs are determined by subtracting the grams of dietary fiber and the grams of sugar alcohols from the grams of total carbohydrates. Dietary fiber does not release insulin into the body. The same is true of sugar alcohols. As a result, you will be able to eat more nutritionally dense foods and may satisfy your food cravings and hunger.

Next, we will look at fats. You will be eating 60 to 75% of your food as fat. This allows for a wide variety of foods, like bacon and pork rinds, to be included in your diet. Avocado, nuts, and other foods will be included in your diet as well. Because you will be eating food that is not processed, it will be important to eat healthy fats including oil derived from natural food sources like avocado oil and coconut oil. High-quality butter and ghee will also be good sources of fat.

When we start to consider proteins, proteins do not need to be lean meats. In fact, the proteins included in keto should not be lean but should be high in fat so that you consume appropriate amounts of fat. The keto diet is only effective when there is a high amount of fat consumed.

Now, let's start calculating the macros. In order to calculate the grams of net carbohydrates to include in your daily diet, it is important to determine your body weight and then your percentage of body fat. To do this, weigh yourself. After determining your weight, divide your body weight by your height in inches and square height in inches squared. Multiply that by 703 and you will have your BMI, or body mass index.

Lbs/height in inches, squared, times 703=BMI. So, in actuality, if you are a 5-foot 6-inch woman weighing 200 lb that's, $200/66^2 \times 703=32.28$. The BMI is 32.28.

Then calculate your body fat percentage. (1.2 x BMI) + (.23 * age) - 5.4 equals body fat percentage. When we plug in the BMI from our female example,

(1.2 * 32.28) + (.23*55) - 5.4 =45.98

So, the body fat percentage is 45.98%. Now that you have your body fat percentage take your body fat percentage and multiply it by your body weight. 45.98% x 200 lb. That equals 91.96 lbs of body fat. Subtract the body fat from your weight and you have your LBM (Lean Body Mass). So, 200 - 91.96 equals 108.04. The LBM is 108.04.

Now, it's time to determine the number of macronutrients to eat each day.
We can start with the calculation for protein. There are .8 grams per pound of lean body mass. In our example, .8* 108.04 equals 84 grams. This is equal to 346 calories

because there are 4 calories in each gram of protein. In our example, 20% of the calories the daily calories will be from protein. Therefore, 346 calories/.20 equals 1730 calories per day.

The total calories are 1730 calories per day.

To determine the number of carbohydrates, let's look at the number of carbohydrates in a gentler keto. 10% of the daily calories will come from carbs. 10% of 1730 calories is 173 calories. If you divide 173 calories by 4 (there are 4 calories in each carbohydrate), you will have 43.25g of carbohydrates as your daily allowance.

The remaining calories for each day will be fat calories:

	346 Calories, Protein
86.50g	20%
	+173 Calories, Carbohydrate
43.25g	10%
	519 Calories of Protein and Carbs
	-1730 (Total Daily Calories)
	1211 Calories, Fat
134.56g	70%

There are 9 calories in each fat gram. 1,211 calories/9 calories = 134.56g of fat for each day, or 70% of your daily calorie intake.

These macros will change as your BMI and LBM change. Make sure you adjust your macros every four or five weeks while you're losing weight so that your macros are accurate. You will want to record what you are eating and review your success in weight loss. This will allow you to track how your body is reacting to food combinations. Each body is different, and it is important to see how you feel when you are eating different foods and combinations of foods as your approach ketosis. Be sure you're eating whole grains and getting fiber through leafy green vegetables. You will also want to be very familiar with nutrition labels to be sure you're not consuming hidden carbohydrates without realizing you are doing so.

Fasting Over 50

Intermittent fasting (IF) is sometimes used to lose weight in combination with a keto diet. It has been an effective way to lose weight for some women. After menopause, some women may gain weight for seemingly no reason. It may be that the general stressors in life cause a new source of weight gain because of cortisol, which may trigger your body to store fat in the abdominal region. Intermittent fasting may be a viable weight loss solution if there is an excess of cortisol being released into your system. The most common forms of IF are 5:2, 12:12, and 16:8.

For the 5:2 fast, one eats normally for 5 days and fasts for 2 days. The two days are not actually a complete fast, but drastically reduced the caloric intake of around 500 calories plus liquids like water and sugar-free drinks. During the 5 days, any foods are allowed to be eaten.

The 12:12 fast is 12 hours of fasting and 12 hours of eating. During the 12 hours of eating, it is important to eat regular meals and snacks. The calorie consumption should be consistent with a normal caloric intake of 2000 recommended calories per day. Make sure the calories are good calories and avoid empty carbohydrates and unhealthy fats.

The same is true for the 16/8 intermediate fast. Fasting lasts for 16 hours. During the 8 hour period, eat at least two meals each day and a snack, maybe two snacks. These meals should be thoughtful meals that do not have excess calories and or carbohydrates.

Fasting, in combination with the keto diet, can promote more rapid weight loss. Fasting may be a way to reach ketosis more quickly. After achieving ketosis, if you've not been intermittently fasting, it may be helpful to introduce fasting to reinitiate weight loss. If you're at a plateau, and you have already been fasting, it may be helpful to begin a different form of fasting. This may trigger new weight loss while in ketosis.

Keto Diet for Longevity

Though there is no absolute proof, recent studies have shown a correlation between the ketogenic diet and a longer, better life. The caveat is, the protein used to replace carbohydrates should be vegetable and plant-based proteins. Additionally, the carbohydrates consumed should be complex. Natural foods are encouraged, and processed carbohydrates, like white bread, sugary carbohydrates and drinks should be avoided. Unhealthy fats should be avoided as well. The fats consumed should be derived from plants to be healthier. This includes avocado oil, olive oil, and coconut oil. The fiber found in bread and other grains eliminated in a keto diet must be replaced with vegetable fiber so that your body continues to be nourished in an appropriate manner. By continuing to eat an appropriate amount of fiber and nutrients, the keto diet can be a healthy and effective weight loss plan.

Some studies are reporting that low-carb diets, including ketogenic diets, are reducing lifespans. The problem with many of these studies is that they are uncontrolled and rely on subjects who report their actions after a period of time has passed. The periods of contact may extend beyond a year or more. To this date, the scientific study of low carbohydrate and ketogenic diets is limited to the study of mice who have been introduced to the ketogenic lifestyle. The mice in the study became less agitated, move about easier, and seem to have better mobility. The lifespan of these mice has also increased.

Overall, it is believed that the improvements in health and evidence of increased longevity through the ketogenic diet are the result of proper study and may be factually true. The reduction of insulin spikes and general weight loss have positive effects on heart health and improve cardiovascular function, especially for people losing weight during and after middle age. With a reduction in inflammation of the body and joints, decreased pain, and increased mobility, people feel better while on the keto diet. Many dieters are able to exercise more as well and are able to exercise on a regular basis. They are able to do all the things people are told will increase their health and lifespan. Health is improved in a way that does go a long way in improving the quality, as well as the longevity of life.

Exercise for Women Over 50 in Support of Keto

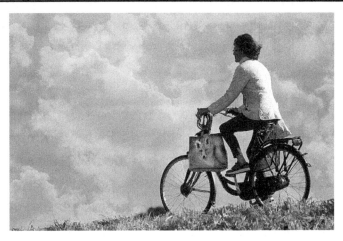

While you are on the keto diet, if your goal is to lose weight, you will be thinking of exercising to assist your body in shedding excess pounds. The problem will be that you may not feel like exercising, especially at the beginning. As your body transitions to ketosis, keto flu may cause feelings of lethargy. When taking all this into account, there are still good reasons for women over the age of 50 to exercise while on the keto diet.

One of the primary reasons exercise is important is the loss of muscle mass women experience as they grow older. In order to combat this loss, exercise is an ideal way to strengthen your body and retain muscle. When we look at what exercises to do, they should be limited, at the beginning of the keto diet, to strengthening and endurance exercises. Even if you are used to strenuous exercise, it is better, until your body adapts to ketosis, to pare down your workouts to a level that does not tire quickly. Your endurance will probably be affected by the switch from using carbs as energy to using fat as energy. It is important not to deplete your energy stores so that your body starts to glean energy from muscles.

As your body enters ketosis, you may find that you feel better, your joints are not as achy, and you're ready to exercise more. Your body is likely to be in better shape than it was, and you will want to capitalize on your new healthy state. This will give you the opportunity to increase your exercises as you enjoy the benefits of the keto diet and ketosis. One should always start out slowly and increase exertion over time so that your muscles are not exhausted and you feel good even while working out. Be sure to drink lots of water during workouts and you may need to replenish nutrients after working out to replace those lost due to sweat and muscle fatigue.

For women over 50, it may be a good idea to limit your exercises to those that do not add a lot of stress to the body. The ability to move around better is often a positive side effect of the keto diet. This will allow you to strengthen and tone your muscles. Start off slowly and add to your exercises as your body recovers and adapts to the keto diet. Be sure to listen to your body as you worked out, and if you feel tired or your muscles feel strained, stop working out for that time period. Your body will tell you how much it can endure.

Switching to a keto diet will cause some strain on your body, to begin with, so take time to build up to a good workout while you are on the diet.

While you're on the keto diet, it will be important to do strength-building exercises and low-intensity workouts in order to continue to burn fat while you're exercising. When you switch over to a high-intensity workout, you will be burning carbohydrates. Because there are only a few carbohydrates in your system, it is difficult to sustain a workout high-intensity level. So, assuming that you are an average person is on the keto diet for weight loss purposes, it will be best to maintain low-intensity workouts. The best are cardio workouts like walking and jogging, as well as strength workouts such as yoga. Yoga is always a good source of exercise as we age. It is a way to strengthen the core and improve balance and muscle tone. If you are using weights in your workout, you should use lighter weights, lighter than you are used to. Increase the repetition so that it is a low-intensity workout. Again, low-intensity workouts burn fat. If weight loss is the goal, you want to lose fat. So, low-intensity exercise should be your goal.

Tips and Tricks for Ketogenic Weight Loss

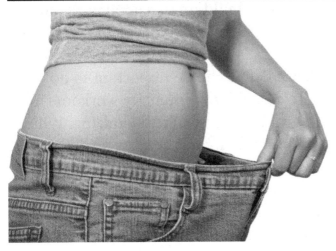

Now that we've gone over the ketogenic diet and all the things involved with being on the ketogenic diet, it is a good time to look at some tips and tips and tricks to being successful on the keto diet.

1. **Limit your carbohydrate intake.** The whole point of the ketogenic diet is to substantially reduce your consumption of carbohydrates. Even if practicing a gentler keto, as recommended for women over 50, you still need to be mindful of the carbs you are consuming. Be sure not to eat hidden carbohydrates that are often found in processed foods. Be wary of "lite" and "low fat" foods. They often get their flavor from sugar. Sugar is, of course, low in fat. On the contrary, sugar is high in carbohydrates. It is a good idea to eliminate almost all forms of sugar on the ketogenic diet. Don't let your carb intake exceed 10%.

2. **Introduce coconut oil into your diet.** Coconut oil is full of nutrients that metabolize quickly in your liver and is converted to energy right away. Consuming coconut oil may help you reach ketosis faster. It's a really easy way to motivate your body to be in ketosis.
3. **Exercise.** It is important to maintain your muscle mass, perhaps increase your muscle mass. Make sure that you're doing exercises involving strength and endurance. Keep the exercises a low-intensity level so that you're burning fat, and not using carbohydrates.
4. **Eat enough fat.** You have to be sure, while you are on the ketogenic diet, that you are eating enough fat. The fat you eat is going to be converted into energy. You need to have enough fat in your body to supply energy to your brain, organs, and muscles to sustain yourself and your activities. Additionally, make sure that you are using your macros to decide what to eat, and that you recalculate your macros from time to time. Be sure you know what you're eating and that you're meeting your nutrient needs, including fat, for each day.
5. **Track your food.** Keep a record of your food consumption. Be sure to add in all the "bits and bites" that pass your lips. You know, the food that you test while cooking? That corner of a cookie you broke off as a little nibble? Record everything you eat so that you know you're meeting your macros. Read labels to make sure you know what you're eating. This book will include a guide on raw foods and meats so that you can calculate how many nutrients are in the foods

that you are eating after you have eliminated processed foods from your diet.
6. **Intermittent fasting.** As previously reviewed in this book, intermittent fasting can be a good way to get into ketosis more quickly. The body will adjust to getting energy from fat molecules in your body, and you may enter ketosis more quickly. You may also use intermittent fasting while you're in ketosis to lose more weight.
7. **Control your protein intake.** If you have been on previous weight loss plans, you are probably adhering to low-fat, high protein diets. Because we are following macros, it is important to eat the correct amount of protein. Do not eat too much protein, because you will throw off your fat or carbohydrates. Eating too little protein will cause your body to lose muscle mass. On the ketogenic diet, we will we want to adhere to the correct ratios of proteins, fats, and carbohydrates in order to optimize weight loss and fat loss in the body.
8. **Drink lots of water.** Water is essential to the body, and you will lose a lot of water on the ketogenic diet. The water must be replaced, especially after exercise. You may also want to take a mineral supplement or drink water with electrolytes so that your chemical balance is maintained after working out. Replacing the water lost through sweat and urination will keep your body working properly. You will feel better if you stay hydrated throughout your ketogenic diet.
9. **Reduce your stress.** Try to remain stress-free during your ketogenic diet. As discussed, cortisol

levels in your body will cause your body to retain fat, especially in the abdominal region. You want to be sure that your body is not working at cross purposes. Stress may trigger your body to store fat in reaction to stress while you are trying to lose fat on your ketogenic diet. Make sure you incorporate activities in your day to reduce your stress level. Some people find yoga is a good way to relax. Others use hobbies as a way to relieve tension and reduce stress.

10. **Get lots of sleep.** Make sure you get enough sleep. Each night your body needs 7 to 9 hours of sleep. Sleep allows us time to rejuvenate our bodies and store up energy. Be sure to do things that promote a sleep-inducing atmosphere. Turn off the lights, limit the use of electronics and like computers and smartphones within 30 minutes of sleeping and refrain from using them in bed. Turn off the television and prepare your room and your body for sleep. Try to maintain a consistent schedule of sleep. These things may make it easier to get to sleep. People on the keto diet have reported better sleep, reduced snoring, and waking up refreshed. Set the scene so that you will be able to benefit from better sleep on the diet.

11. **Know your goals.** Before you start the ketogenic diet, determine your goals, and write down the reasons why you're on the ketogenic diet. If you want to lose weight, also note why you want to lose weight. This is important, so you can always refer back to the reasons you began the diet. It is sometimes helpful to remember what your goals are and why you want to

meet those goals. This will be a good touchstone when you want to reach for a cookie or a sugary drink. Make sure you have that goal handy so that when you're feeling weak, you can remind yourself of your goals are and be determined to stick to them.

Chapter 3: Keto Food and Ketosis

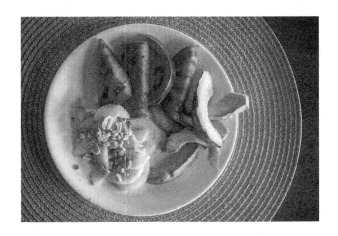

After determining what the macros look like and how many calories you should be consuming each day, you will need to decide what to eat. There are many options that are keto-friendly, so finding something to eat will probably not be a problem. There will have to be decisions made regarding food quality and food quantity.

Food Quality

It is better to eat foods that are of high quality on the keto diet. The right chemical makeup of your food assists in a successful journey to ketosis. Because you will be using food to fuel your body, it is important to eat the best quality food available to get the key nutrients you will need to sustain your brain and body health.

Grass-fed meat from grazing animals is suggested because it tends to be higher in omega-3 fatty acids. Cage-free poultry and eggs are also preferred on keto. Butter should be of high quality with high-fat content. Grass-fed meats clan to have fewer calories than grain-fed needs. Additionally, the grain-fed to conventionally bred animals often contains growth hormone which will be passed to you when you eat it. The grass-fed meat products are healthier and lower in calories. There can be up to five times more omega-3 fatty acids in grass-fed beef than grain-fed. Grass-fed beef also contains electrolytes. Electrolytes control nerve pulses and muscle contractions. They leave your body through urination, which will be more frequent while on the keto diet. Electrolytes need to be replaced to keep your body in balance. Grass-fed beef will help to restore magnesium, potassium, and sodium and assist in minimizing the effects of the keto flu.

Eating organic vegetables and fruit, though not required, may be considered optimal when you are making an effort to eat the cleanest and healthiest food. Whether an item is organic or conventional, the keto effects are the same. The benefit of eating organic food is a reduction in the amount of chemicals and pesticide residue. The nutritional characteristics are the same and hold true whether the produce is fresh or frozen. No matter what, be sure to cleanse your produce and your preparation area regularly. Inspect the produce for pests and debris to be sure the washing and soaking have done a good job, especially when you are eating raw fruits and vegetables. Remember to concentrate on dark green vegetables and try to get the freshest possible. Good quality produce will provide good nutrients to fuel your body.

Foods to Eat

The variety of foods you can eat on the keto diet is vast. After determining the macros to follow, you can find foods that fit into the macros for your daily food. It will be important to have enough nutrients to sustain yourself while on the diet and to be able to safely stay on the keto diet.

Fats

Your daily consumption of fats will be around 70% of your food intake. This needs to be high-quality fat that stays in your system to be used as energy. These are typically found in fats that are the result of raw foods and animals.

Some of the best fats for keto are:

Hard Cheeses
Nuts like almonds, walnuts, pecans, and macadamia
Seeds from sunflowers, pumpkins, chia, flaxseed and hemp hearts
Natural oils like olive oil and coconut oil
Cacao of at least 85% cacao. This must be unsweetened and unprocessed chocolate
Poultry, especially dark meat
Fatty fish
Whole eggs, especially the yolks
Whole milk produces like whole milk mozzarella and ricotta

Cheese

When we look at high-fat foods, cheese tops the list. It is high in fat and has no carbohydrates. Unfortunately, cheese contains a lot of calories, along with unhealthy saturated fats. When you are consuming cheese, be mindful of the amount you eat. Some cheese is a healthy snack and a good alternative to chips and sugary snack items. Small amounts of cheese in your diet, a few ounces daily, will help you control your hunger because it is filling. It has also been found that calcium in cheese may have a positive effect on blood pressure and cholesterol. Consumption of cheese has also been found to increase muscle mass.

Nuts

As you choose which nuts you're going to eat on keto, be sure to take note of the net carbs. Some nuts have more fat than others, and some have more calories and carbohydrates than others. Choose nuts that will fit well in your macros. Because of the high calories and carbs eat nuts in moderation. They may also have a significant amount of protein when eating a large quantity. Be sure you are adhering to your protein macros as well as your carbohydrate macros.

Seeds

The good thing about seeds in relation to keto is that the carbohydrates are mostly offset by fiber. That makes the net carbohydrates friendly for keto. Seeds tend to be high in fat and contain some protein. They often contain harmful omega-6 fatty acids, though. You can benefit from the healthy concentration of nutrients in seeds, but eating them sprouted. In order to sprout seeds, simply germinate the seeds between two wet paper towels and leave them to sit for 2 to 8 days. Make sure your paper towel remains moist. Eventually, the stem will sprout from the seed. It's still high in nutrients but easier to digest.

Oils

Oils can be your best cooking aid in the keto diet. They must be able to burn at high temperatures to be most effective for cooking. It is important to use unsaturated fats to provide the most heart-healthy oils. The polyunsaturated oils will be a good addition to the fats consumed on a keto like nut oils and avocado oils. These will assist you in achieving a healthy, effective keto diet. Avocado oil, sesame oil, coconut oil, and olive oil have essential qualities to aid in digestion and nutrient absorption. Also, coconut oil speeds up metabolism.

Meat/Fish/Eggs/Dairy

Unprocessed meats do not contain carbohydrates, and many are high in fat. Grass-fed meats are better than grain-fed but watch the portion size. Be careful not to exceed the protein requirements in your daily macros. Fish is good, especially fish high in fat like salmon. Avoid the breading, which has carbohydrates. Again, wild-caught fish is better. It is fed naturally off of foods fish are accustomed to eating. This is Lloyd's the chance that growth hormones and antibiotics may be included in the feed from farm fat raised fish. Along the same lines, try to stick to cage-free pasture-raised eggs in the hopes of avoiding chemical additives that might reduce the quality of the food you are consuming. The same is true for milk. Milk and dairy products should be organic to avoid growth hormones and antibiotics that may be found in conventional Foods today. Meat fish eggs and dairy are high in fat; I can be a good source of the fat you need to consume on the keto diet.

Proteins

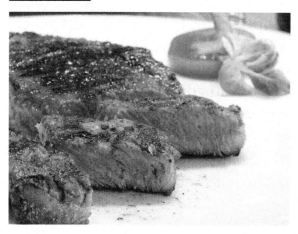

Protein will make up 20% of your daily food intake. It is important not to exceed your protein macros. Be sure you're making good decisions regarding your protein if a person that you are including your diet. It will be consuming a lot of fat, which may contain a lot of protein. So you have to be sure to combine your fat macros with your protein macros when you're setting up your meal plan for the day.

Some of the proteins that you will be eating that are most

efficient are:

Salmon
Mackerel
Tuna
Sardines
Eggs
Greek yogurt
Shrimp
Chicken thighs
Peanuts
Pistachios
Almonds
Soybeans (edamame)
Nut butters

The goal of the keto diet is not to eat low-fat proteins. Luckily, there are many high-fat proteins available for consumption. Many times, you will be able to satisfy your fat macros and protein macros with the same food items. Watch your calories, and be sure to incorporate your snack foods into your protein count. Be mindful that green leafy vegetables also contain protein.

It is important to consume enough protein so that carbohydrates in your body do not use muscle to convert to energy. Conversely, too much protein can cause muscle tissue to break down and turn into sugar because of the lack of carbohydrates available on a low-carb diet. Eat the right amount of protein, and don't forget about adding in the protein found snacks and vegetables, especially cream leafy ones when considering your protein macros.

Fish

Some of the best foods for protein on keto are fatty proteins found in salmon, mackerel, and sardines. These proteins are high in fat and omega-3 fatty acids. Fresh fish is higher in omega-3 fatty acid than canned fish, but if you are going to eat fish protein, make sure it is high in fat. This is an efficient way to consume protein and fat that will be converted to energy.

Eggs

Some studies indicate that people who include dairy in their diet have less hunger, and the consumption of dairy may inhibit the production of cortisol, and therefore, the resulting abdominal fat. Full-fat dairy is high in calories, so be sure not to over-consume. It is common for conventional milk and dairy products to contain growth hormones. Dairy from grass-fed animals and organic dairy products are recommended. Aside from the hormones, conventional dairy products do not have as high levels of omega-3 fatty acids, which have anti-inflammatory qualities and promote joint health. Dairy contains a lot of protein. If you're eating meat protein, you should be especially cognizant of the amount of dairy that you're eating so you do not exceed your protein macros. Egg whites are lower in calories and contain the protein of the egg. The egg yolks contain the fat of eggs. If you're going to eat meat and eggs and you have consumed enough fat for the daily macro, you may be able to eat the white instead of the yolks without adding additional fat. The yolk also carries the bulk of calories from eggs and egg whites have very few calories.

Nuts/Nut Butters/Soybeans

Nuts and soybeans (edamame) make excellent snack foods on keto. Eating good quality protein and protein-filled snacks, especially after exercising, may assist your body in building muscle. Snacks should be kept small. They should simply be a means to curb your hunger pains. That is why a quick snack of nuts is ideal. They contain some proteins, some fats, and some carbohydrates. Count the nuts you select to be sure you don't eat too many carbs. Carefully measure the serving size of your snack. Since nuts are small, it is easy to think that eating a few extra nuts here and there won't matter. Whether this is true depends on the nut. That's a good way to add moderate levels of protein to your diet and to adjust your protein macros for the day.

Carbohydrates

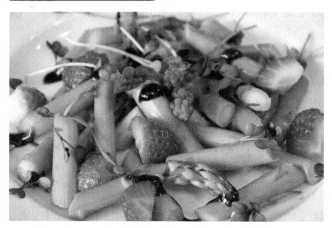

So far, it has been stressed to eat more fat, the correct amount of protein, and now, it is time for carbohydrates. Eat fewer carbohydrates. Consume 10% of your daily food in the form of carbohydrates. This is the crux of the ketogenic diet. Normally, carbohydrates are limited to 5% of the daily calories eaten. In doing the gentle keto, the carbohydrates are increased to 10%. Whether 5% or 10%, be sure to minimize the number of carbohydrates in your diet. Also, try to make the carbohydrates of good quality that will burn off quickly so that your body moves quickly to burning fat.

There are many no-carb options available when eating fats and protein. What is needed to add to your diet are vegetables. Produce has nutrients and vitamins that your body needs, so they should be included in your diet. Be sure to incorporate foods that have valuable nutrients such as vegetables and berries into your diet. These are low in carbohydrates. Some of the vegetables and fruits should be used more sparingly than others. Look at green leafy vegetables and vegetables that grow above the ground as low carbohydrate options to provide healthy options that will not add fat. Vegetables that grow underground like carrots and potatoes tend to have more sugar content and are higher in carbohydrates. Here is a list of fruits and vegetables that are good to eat on keto (Yes), should be excluded from your keto diet (No), and fruits and vegetables that may be eaten occasionally (Maybe):

Yes	**No**	**Maybe**
Asparagus	Apples	Artichokes
Avocado	Apricots	Blackberries
Bell peppers	Bananas	Blueberries
Bok choy	Beets	Broccoli
Broccoli rabe	Cantaloupe	Brussels sprouts

Cauliflower	Cherries	Carrots
Celery	Corn	Coconut meat
Cucumbers	Cranberries	Eggplant
Greens	Dried fruit	Fennel
Mushrooms	Grapes	Ginger
Radishes	Leek	Honeydew
Sprouts (alfalfa, bean)	Mango	Jicama
Summer squash (zucchini, yellow)	Oranges	Kiwi
	Papaya	Lemon juice
	Peaches	Lime juice

	Pears	Olives (black, green)
YES	**NO**	**Maybe**
	Pineapple	Onions
	Plums	Raspberries
	Potatoes	Rhubarb
	Sweet potatoes	Spaghetti Squash
	Watermelon	Strawberries
	Winter Squash	Tomatoes

Green leafy vegetables like kale, spinach, collard greens, mustard greens, romaine lettuce, and arugula are low in net carbohydrates and high in vitamins and nutrients. These items should be integrated into your keto diet so that you are sure to be receiving enough nutrients for a healthy diet. Though not "free" foods, because they have carbohydrates of varying amounts, they are items that you can eat easily and are necessary for soluble fibers. Eating your vegetables may help to stave off constipation. Leafy greens and other vegetables where you eat the parts of the plant exposed to pesticides are better if purchased organic. If you do not purchase organically-grown products, be sure to clean your leafy greens, even if it is packaged and says it is pre-washed.

The items in the "NO" column are very high in sugar and carbohydrates. Eating them will easily knock you out of ketosis. Even though some of the items are vegetables, root vegetables have a lot of sugar. Also, most fruits are not allowed on keto.

Avocados are also in the carbohydrate section of foods. Basically, avocados are the keto superfood. They are high in fat and protein, low in carbohydrates. They have good nutritional value.

The only fruits that are really allowed on the keto diet are berries. Because you eat the seed, they are higher in fiber. They tend to be the lowest carbohydrates in the fruit families. Avocados are a nice addition because they are high in fat and high in fiber, as well as low in carbohydrates. Other fruits are very high in sugar. In fact, two apples can be your entire carbohydrate macro for a day.

If you feel you need to eat starchy, Foods replace those foods with cauliflower. Cauliflower has two grams of net carbs per cup. Potatoes have 26 grams per cup and rice has 45 grams per cup. These carb counts have been a reason for the increasing popularity of riced cauliflower. Luckily, it is available frozen and packaged in the fresh produce section of most grocery stores, so its not necessary to waste time operating your food processor.

Some other vegetables that you may eat on your keto diet are asparagus, green beans, mushrooms, tomatoes, eggplant, cucumber, bell pepper, celery, and cabbage. Onions are also included on the keto diet mainly because they are eaten sparingly, and the amount of onions in a recipe is spread out among many servings in a dish.

Adding a variety of vegetables into your keto diet may help you to feel better and also help you avoid some of the negative effects of the keto diet like constipation and possibly the keto flu. It is important to maintain adequate vitamins and nutrients in your diet, and vegetables and berries fit the bill. Vegetables such as spinach, kale, collard greens, turnip greens, romaine lettuce, and certain cabbages are foods that you can eat without affecting ketosis. They are high in nutrients and low in net carbs.

Below is a generalized list of foods and their nutritional content. Check the entire nutritional content of foods and maintain the correct serving sizes, so you do not exceed the calories allowed with your keto macros.

Nutritional Food List

Food	Serving	Net Car	Protein	Fat	Calories

	Size	b			
Alfalfa sprouts	1/2 cup	1g	1.5g	0g	15
Almond butter (w/o salt)	1 Tbls	1.5g	3.5g	9g	98
Almond meal/flour	1/4 cup	3g	6g	11g	150
Almonds	23 nuts	2.5g	6g	14g	164
Artichoke	1/2 medium	3.5g	1.7g	0g	32
Artichoke hearts, canned	1 heart	0.5g	0g	1.5g	15
Food	**Serving Size**	**Net Carb**	**Protein**	**Fat**	**Calories**
Artichoke hearts, marinated	4 pieces	2g	0g	6g	60

Arugula	1 cup	0.5g	0.5g	0g	5
Asparagus	6 spears	2g	2g	0g	20
Avocado	1/2 fruit	3.5g	3.5g	15g	182
Bamboo shoots	1/2 cup	1g	1g	0g	12
Beans, green	1/2 cup	2g	1g	0g	16
Beet greens	1/2 cup	2g	2g	0g	19
Blackberries, fresh	1/4 cup	4g	0.5g	0.2g	15
Blackberries, frozen	1/4 cup	4g	0.5g	0.2g	24
Blue cheese	1 oz.	0.7g	6g	8g	100
Bok choy	1/2 cup	0.5g	1.3g	0g	10

Food	Serving Size	Net Carb	Protein	Fat	Calories
Boston/bibb lettuce	1 cup	0g	1g	0g	7
Brazil nuts	5 nuts	1g	3.5g	17g	165
Brie	1 oz.	0.1g	6g	8g	95
Broccoflower	1/2 cup	1g	1g	0g	10
Broccoli	1/2 cup	3g	2g	0g	27
Food	**Serving Size**	**Net Carb**	**Protein**	**Fat**	**Calories**
Broccoli florets	1/2 cup	1g	1g	0g	10
Broccoli rabe	1/2 cup	0.3g	3.3g	0.5g	28
Brussels sprouts	1/4 cup	2g	1g	0g	14
Butter or ghee	1 Tbls	0g	0.12g	11.5g	102

Cabbage, green	1/2 cup	2.5g	1g	0g	17
Cabbage, red	1/2 cup	3g	1g	0g	22
Cabbage, savoy	1/2 cup	2g	1.3g	0g	17
Cashew butter (w/o salt)	1 Tbls	4g	3g	8g	94
Cashews	1/4 cup	9g	4g	12g	150
Cauliflower	1/2 cup	1g	1g	0.3g	14
Cauliflower florets	1/2 cup	2g	1g	0g	13
Celery	1 stalk	0.5g	0g	0g	6
Celery	1/2 cup	1.8g	0.5g	0g	14
Chard, swiss	1/2 cup	1.5g	2g	0g	18

Food	Serving Size	Net Carb	Protein	Fat	Calories
Chayote	1/2 cup	2g	0.5g	0.4g	19
Cheddar or colby	1 oz.	1g	6.5g	9.5g	115
Cherries, fresh, pitted	1/4 cup	5g	0.4g	0.1g	24
Chicory greens	½ cup	0.5g	0g	0g	3
Chinese cabbage	1/2 cup	0.5g	0.5g	0g	5
Chives	1 Tbls	0g	0.1g	0g	1
Coconut, shredded, unsweetened	1/4 cup	1g	1g	7g	71
Coconut butter	1 Tbls	1.5g	1g	10.5g	105
Coconut oil	1 Tbls	0g	0g	13.47g	121

Food	Servi	Net	Protei	Fat	Calori
Collard greens	1/2 cup	1.5g	2.5g	1g	31
Cottage cheese (2% fat)	1/2 cup	5g	12g	2.5g	92
Cranberries, raw, chopped	1/4 cup	2g	0.1g	0g	13
Cream cheese	2 Tbls	0.6g	2g	10g	100
Cucumber (with peel)	1/2 cup, sliced	1.7g	0.3g	0g	8
Daikon radish	1/2 cup	1g	0.4g	0g	9
Dandelion greens	1/2 cup	2g	1g	0.3g	17
Eggplant	1/2 cup	3g	1g	0g	17
Endive	1/2 cup	0g	0.3g	0g	4

	ng Size	Carb	n		es
Escarole	1/2 cup	0.3g	1g	0g	14
Fennel, bulb	1/2 cup	1.5g	0.5g	0g	13
Fennel, bulb	1/2 cup	2g	0.5g	0g	13
Flaxseed oil	1 Tbls	0g	0.01g	13.6g	120
Goat cheese (soft)	1 oz.	0g	5g	6g	75
Gouda	1 oz.	0.6g	7g	8g	100
Greens, mixed	1 cup	0.5g	0.5g	0g	5
Hazelnuts	12 nuts	1.5g	2.5g	10g	106
Hearts of palm	1 heart	0.5g	1g	0.2g	9
Heavy whipping	1 Tbls	0.4g	0.4g	5.4g	51

Food	Serving Size	Net Carb	Protein	Fat	Calories
cream					
Heavy whipping cream	1/2 cup	1.6g	1.7g	22g	204
Iceberg lettuce	1 cup	1g	0.7g	0g	10
Jicama	1/2 cup	2g	0.5g	0g	23
Kale	1/2 cup	2.5g	1g	0g	18
Kohlrabi	1/4 cup	2.5g	1g	0g	12
Lard/Dripping	1 Tbls	0g	0g	12.8g	115
Food	**Serving Size**	**Net Carb**	**Protein**	**Fat**	**Calories**
Leeks	1/2 cup	3.5g	0.5g	0g	16
Loganberries, frozen	1/4 cup	3g	0.6g	0.1g	20

Loose-leaf lettuce	1 cup	2g	0.5g	0g	8
Macadamia butter	1 Tbls	1g	2g	10g	97
Macadamias	6 nuts	0.8g	1g	11g	102
Mayonnaise	1 Tbls	0.08g	0.13g	10.33g	94
Melon, cantaloupe	1/4 cup	3g	0.4g	0.1g	15
Melon, honeydew	1/4 cup	3.5g	0.2g	0.1g	16
Mozzarella (whole milk)	1 oz.	0.6g	6.3g	6.3g	85
Mung bean sprouts	1/2 cup	2g	1.5g	0g	16
Mushrooms, white	1/4 cup	1g	1g	0g	11
Mushrooms, shiitake	1/4 cup	4g	0.5g	0g	20

Food	Serving Size	Net Carb	Protein	Fat	Calories
Mustard greens	1/2 cup	1.5g	2g	0.3g	18
Nopales (cactus pads)	1/2 cup	1g	1g	0g	11
Okra	1/2 cup	1.5g	1.5g	0g	18
Olive oil	1 Tbls	0g	0g	13.5g	119

Food	Serving Size	Net Carb	Protein	Fat	Calories
Olives, black	5	1g	0g	3g	30
Olives, green	5	0.1g	0g	2g	20
Onion, chopped	2 Tbls	1.5g	0.2g	0g	8
Parmesan	1 oz.	1g	10g	7.3g	111
Parsley	1 Tbls	0.1g	0.1g	0g	1
Pecans	10 halves	0.5g	1.3g	10g	98

Peppers, green bell	1/2 cup	2g	1g	0g	15
Peppers, green bell	1/4 cup	0.5g	0g	3.5g	37
Peppers, red bell	1/2 cup	3g	1g	0g	23
Peppers, red bell	1/4 cup	1.5g	0.3g	3.5g	35
Pine nuts	2 Tbls	0.7g	2.7g	14g	148
Pistachios	25 nuts	3g	3.5g	8g	98
Pumpkin	1/4 cup	2g	0.5g	0g	12
Pumpkin seeds (hulled)	1/4 cup	1g	9g	14g	180
Radicchio	1/2 cup	0.8g	0.3g	0g	5
Radishes	6	0.2g	0g	0g	2

Food	Serving Size	Net Carb	Protein	Fat	Calories
Raspberries, fresh	1/4 cup	3.5g	0.4g	0.2g	16
Raspberries, frozen	1/4 cup	2g	0.4g	0.2g	18
Ricotta (whole milk)	1/2 cup	4g	14g	16g	216
Romaine lettuce	1 cup	0.5g	0.5g	0g	8
Sauerkraut	1/2 cup	1g	0.7g	0g	13
Scallion/green onion	1/4 cup	1g	0.5g	0g	8
Sesame seed oil	1 Tbls	0g	0g	13.6g	120
Sesame seeds	2 Tbls	2g	3.2g	9g	103
Shallots	2 Tbls	3g	0.5g	0g	14

Food	Serving Size	Net Carb	Protein	Fat	Calories
Sour cream	1 Tbls	0.6g	0.3g	2.3g	24
Spaghetti squash	1/2 cup	4g	0.5g	0g	21
Spinach	1 cup	0.3g	1g	0g	7
Spinach	1/2 cup	1g	3g	0g	21
Strawberries, fresh, sliced	1/4 cup	2g	0.3g	0.2g	13
Strawberries, frozen	1/4 cup	2.5g	0.2g	0g	13
Strawberry, fresh	1 large	1g	0.1g	0.1g	6
Food	**Serving Size**	**Net Carb**	**Protein**	**Fat**	**Calories**
Summer squash	1/2 cup	2.5g	1g	0.4g	21
Sunflower seed butter	1 Tbls	3g	2.8g	9g	99

Sunflower seeds (hulled)	1/4 cup	3g	6g	15g	160
Swiss cheese	1 oz.	0.4g	7.6g	9g	111
Tahini (sesame paste)	1 Tbls	2g	2.6g	8g	89
Tomato	1 small	2.5g	1g	0g	16
Tomato	1/4 cup	2g	0.5g	0g	11
Tomato	1 medium	3.5g	1g	0.25g	22
Tomato, cherry	5	2.3g	1g	0.2g	15
Turnips	1/2 cup	3.5g	1g	0g	25
Walnut oil	1 Tbls	0g	0g	13.6	120
Walnuts	7 halves	1g	2g	9g	93

Watercress	1/2 cup	0.1g	0.4g	0g	2
Yogurt (plain unsweetened/whole milk)	1/2 cup	5.3	4g	3.7g	69
Zucchini	1/2 cup	1.5g	1g	0.3g	14

Spices and Sauces for Flavor

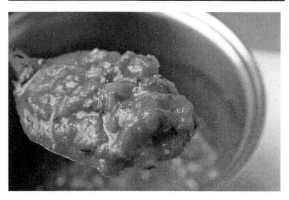

Because of the restrictions of the keto diet, sauces like ketchup and barbecue sauce have too much sugar and too many carbohydrates to include on your food list. Fortunately, most herbs have minimal amounts of carbohydrates. Spices have a little more carbs, but not so many that they are prohibited from the diet plan.

Here is a list of spices and herbs with nutritional information is based on 1teaspoon of herbs or spices.

NAME	NET CARBS	PROTEIN	FAT	CALORIES
Basil Leaves, Dried	2.21	1.09	0.19	11
Basil Leaves, Fresh	0.04	0.15	0.03	1.17
Bay Leaves, Dried	2.29	0.36	0.4	14.83
Black Pepper, Ground	1.82	0.49	0.15	11.83
Caraway Seed	0.56	0.93	0.69	15.67
Cardamom	1.92	0.51	0.32	14.67
Cayenne Pepper, Ground	1.39	0.57	0.82	15
Celery Flakes, Dried	1.69	0.53	0.1	15
Celery Seed	1.4	0.85	1.19	18.5
Chili Powder	0.7	0.64	0.68	13.33
Chives, Dried	1.81	1	0.17	14.67

NAME	NET CARBS	PROTEIN	FAT	CALORIES
Chives, Fresh	0.09	0.16	0.04	1.5
Cilantro, Dried	1.98	1.04	0.23	13.17
Cilantro, Fresh	0.04	0.1	0.03	1.17
Cinnamon, Ground	1.29	0.19	0.06	11.67
Clove, Ground	1.5	0.28	0.62	13
Coriander Seed	0.62	0.59	0.84	14
Coriander, Dried	1.98	1.04	0.23	13.17
Cumin Seed	1.59	0.84	1.05	17.67
Cumin, Ground	1.59	0.84	1.05	17.67
Curry Powder	0.12	0.68	0.66	15.33
Dill Weed, Dried	1.99	0.94	0.21	12
Dill Weed, Fresh	0.23	0.16	0.05	2
Fennel Seed	0.59	0.75	0.7	16.33
Garlic Powder	3	0.78	0.04	15.67

NAME	NET CARBS	PROTEIN	FAT	CALORIES
Ginger Root, Fresh	0.74	0.09	0.04	3.83
Ginger, Ground	2.72	0.43	0.2	15.83
Horseradish	0.21	0.03	0.02	1.21
Lemongrass, Fresh	1.2	0.09	0.02	4.67
Marjoram, Dried	0.96	0.6	0.33	12.83
Mustard, Ground	0.74	1.23	1.71	24
Nutmeg, Ground	1.35	0.28	1.72	24.83
Onion Powder	3.02	0.49	0.05	16.17
Oregano, Dried	1.26	0.43	0.2	12.5
Paprika, Ground	0.9	0.67	0.61	13.33
Parsley, Dried	1.13	1.26	0.26	13.83
Parsley, Fresh	0.015	0.14	0.04	1.67
Peppermint, Fresh	0.32	0.18	0.05	3.33

Poppy Seed	0.41	0.85	1.96	24.83
Red Pepper, Ground	1.39	0.57	0.82	15
Rosemary, Dried	1.01	0.23	0.72	15.67
Rosemary, Fresh	0.31	0.16	0.28	6.17
Saffron	2.91	0.54	0.28	14.67
Sage, Ground	0.97	0.5	0.6	14.83
Salt	0	0	0	0
Tarragon, Dried	2.02	1.08	0.34	14
Thyme, Dried	1.3	0.43	0.35	13
Thyme, Fresh	0.49	0.26	0.08	4.83
Turmeric Root	0.13	0.02	0.03	1.17
Turmeric, Ground	2.11	0.46	0.15	14.67
White Pepper, Ground	2.01	0.49	0.1	14

Since there are carbohydrates in most of the herbs and spices and calories as well, measure what you are adding to your food and count the amounts in your macros. The same is true for condiments. Below are the carb counts for low-carb condiments that fit into the keto diet.

FOOD	SERVING SIZE	NET CARBS (G)
Dressings, creamy (ranch, blue cheese, Caesar, etc.)	2 tbsp	2
Dressings, oil or vinaigrette	2 tbsp	2.7
Hot sauce (sriracha, buffalo, red pepper sauce, etc.)	1 tsp	1.2
FOOD	SERVING SIZE	NET CARBS (G)
Lemon juice, lime juice	2 tbsp	2.5
Marinara sauce	1/2 cup	7.4
Mayonnaise	1 tbsp	0.1
Mustard	1 tsp	0.1
Pesto sauce	1/4 cup	2.8
Salsa	2 tbsp	1.7
Vinegar – balsamic	1 tbsp	2.7

| Vinegar – white, apple cider | 1 tbsp | 0 |

What Foods to Avoid

For the low carb portion of the diet, avoid grains, fruits with high sugar content, starchy vegetables, fruit juice and carrot juice, sugar (including honey and syrup), chips, crackers, and baked goods. These items are high in sugar and/or carbohydrates and will not be useful in a low-carbohydrate diet.

Fruits and Starchy Vegetables - Juice, fruit, and sugar are definite no-nos on the keto diet. The excess sugars will not only spike your carbohydrates, but they will also cause insulin to be released in response to the spike in blood sugar. This is all the opposite of the goal of ketosis. There will be too many carbohydrates available for the body to convert to energy. This will make it impossible for the body to be starved of carbs and glucose and the body will not switch to using fat as energy. Starchy vegetables like corn and beets have high sugar content. Bananas, apples, raisins, and mangoes are too high in sugar content to include on the keto diet. Fruit and sugar will have to be avoided to reach ketosis.

Grains, Bread, and Pasta - Grains are high in carbohydrates. Don't try to substitute grains with gluten-free bread and pasta. Even the gluten-free items tend to replace the grains with other foods that are also high in carbohydrates like chickpea flour. To replace pasta, try the zucchini spirals or shirataki noodles. These noodles are very low in carbohydrates and may be an alternative to high carb grain pasta that meets your needs. Butternut squash spirals are also readily available, but winter squash is high in carbohydrates. Quinoa is a protein-rich grain; there are too many carbohydrates for this grain to be included in the keto food list. Rice and potatoes, brown rice and sweet potatoes have too many carbs for even the healthy alternatives to be included in your food plan.

Legumes - Avoid beans and legumes like lentils, pinto, black beans, and chickpeas. Though they happen to be high in fiber, they unfortunately also are high in carbohydrates. That makes beans a poor addition to the ketogenic diet. They can be used sparingly when added in small amounts to recipes like soups and stews. They are nutritious, but like starchy vegetables, they do not fit well in the keto lifestyle.

Coated Meat -Meats with added sugar such as maple flavored sausage and bacon should be avoided. Also, breaded chicken and fish are not allowed on the keto diet. These foods have carbohydrates and are not options on the diet. It is better to eat food that is less processed, and if there are any added flavorings, you should add them yourself to maintain control of the additions.

Low Fat - Foods labeled as low fat often contain sugar or unapproved sugar substitutes, which act like sugar and trick your body into a spike in blood sugar and short term satisfaction. This is true for items you may not associate with sweet flavors like salad dressing and mayonnaise. In these instances, full-fat options are included on the keto diet so it's okay to eat the real food and avoid processed imitation.

Vegetable Oils - The nutritional value of vegetable, canola, and corn oils are not ideal for the keto diet. They like the nutritional values of higher quality oils and are high in polyunsaturated fatty acids (PUFA). These PUFAs are bad for your heart as they release plaque into arteries. They also cause inflammation in the liver and may promote liver disease. In fact, vegetable oils may be a cause of obesity. Vegetable oil is unhealthy.

Of course, most foods are technically allowed on the ketogenic diet. In order to include some of these forbidden foods in your diet and remain in ketosis, measure your foods and flavorings and know what you are consuming when it comes to carbohydrates and overall calories. Because the consumption of carbohydrates spikes blood sugar levels, when blood sugar drops, there will be a feeling of malaise and hunger when the carbohydrates wear off. It is better to eat more calories from foods that will sustain a constant level of blood sugar and foods that will help keep your stomach feeling full.

Keto Approved Sweeteners

On this very low carb diet, sugar and sweetener are eliminated. There is no room in the diet for sugar-based carbohydrates. Fortunately, there are substitutes that can be used in place of sugar if you are baking keto items or even to add to coffee or tea. The best sweeteners on keto are stevia and erythritol. These can be used independently or combined.

There are several sweeteners that are keto-friendly:

Sweetener	Measure	Type	Net Carbs	Calories
Stevia	1/2 Cup	Natural	5	20
Monk Fruit	1/2 Cup	Natural	25	100
Erythritol	1/2 Cup	Sugar Alcohol	5	20
Sucralose	1/2 Cup	Artificial	0	0
Aspartame	1/2 Cup	Artificial	85	352
Saccharin	1/2 Cup	Artificial	94	364
Table Sugar	1/2 Cup	Processed	100	387

Stevia and erythritol are both plant-based sweeteners that can be used in place of sugar and but with drastically fewer calories. Stevia three times sweeter than sugar, erythritol is nearly twice as sweet as sugar. Because they are sweeter than sugar, it is not necessary to use as much of the sweeteners are you would use sugar. Stevia is a plant, the leaves of which are naturally sweet. Stevia is available in powder form, granulated and liquid form.

Erythritol is derived from plants, as well. The plants must be processed and the sweetness is extracted through a fermentation of plant leaves when sugar alcohols are extracted. The resulting sugar alcohol can be up to 80% sweeter than regular sugar. Erythritol is only available in granulated form. Erythritol is not absorbed completely by the body. This is one of the reasons it fits into the keto diet. Because it is not completely absorbed, it does not greatly affect insulin production.

Both stevia and erythritol can be used in baking on a keto diet. The two artificial sweeteners do not melt as quickly as regular sugar, so there may be some modifications necessary for successful baking. Since they are both commercially prepared, it may be that additives affect the number of carbs in the finished product in an effort to produce a consistent product.

Keto on a Budget

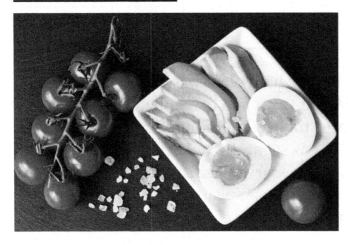

One of the things that people say against the keto diet is that it is expensive. In reality, it doesn't have to be expensive. You can do the keto diet for the same amount of money as any other food plan. The recommendations for grass-fed beef and organic produce are recommendations. It's true that grass-fed beef is healthier. But you will be able to reach ketosis without grass-fed meat. Some of the items are more expensive, that is just a fact. But you are investing in yourself, and you are worth it. While you may be spending more money on your food that you're purchasing, you will also be saving money on food that you previously purchased but no longer suits your lifestyle. There will be no more sugary snacks, no more potato chips. These items cost a lot of money as well. By eating fresh foods, you will be saving yourself money.

So, if you're on a budget doing keto, the first thing you should do is to try to locate items on the diet at a lower cost. Be sure to see what you can find on the internet. Look for items in retail stores in your area that you know are less expensive than other stores. Organic products and grass-fed meats are available in most communities. They are more expensive, but you may be able to find them at a lower price at different locations. This is especially true if you seek out some of the items on the internet.

Though organic products are easy to find, one of the main advantages of the keto diet is that its not necessary to eat organic produce, and you don't have to ingest grass-fed meats. You do want to get the best quality that you can.

When you're addressing your diet, you may just be moving your food dollars from one category of food to another category of food. In other words, some foods that you are used to buying may fall off your list entirely. Also, it is not necessary to purchase prepackaged ketogenic foods. These products are manufactured for a variety of diets, and many times, they just put a keto-friendly label on the box to sell it. These foods may contain more carbohydrates than you want to consume. Remember, there are several kinds of keto diets. What may work on one keto diet may not work for your keto diet. Besides, since you will be preparing many meals, you can add snack bars and snack foods to your ketogenic baking repertoire. The keto snacks are typically expensive. By making the snacks yourself, you will be saving money and controlling what nutrients you include in your diet.

You can use your food dollars to be creative with food, and if you are accustomed to not preparing your own food, you may find that you're saving money in the long run by not consistently eating out. Just like any other budget item, there is usually a way to work around restrictions of your budget. You can be on the keto diet without breaking your budget by purchasing items in bulk like nuts and flours. The internet offers a lot of opportunities to save money while you're on the keto diet. Stay away from processed foods even keto-friendly foods. It is very possible to be on the ketogenic diet without spending more money. When you eliminate processed foods from your budget, you end up with fresh foods and you control your intake of those foods. It may be necessary to plan a menu and use your menu to determine your grocery list. In the end, you may end up saving money because you only purchase what is on your list and staples for your pantry. You may find that you are not spending more money even if you purchase grass-fed meats and organic products. This is because impulse buys are eliminated and you stick to what you need and do not purchase items that are extraneous to your budget.

Keto Away From Home

The ketogenic diet needs to travel with you no matter where you are. At times you may need to go to parties or may want to go to parties and gatherings, and you may fear the temptations of food items at the party. One way to eliminate the worry is to prepare something and take it with you to the party. If you bring an item for everyone to enjoy, you will be providing a hostess gift as well as a dish that you know you can eat. That way you will not be stuck eating crudités and drinking water. You will be able to prepare an item that you enjoy and that others will enjoy with you.

If you are friendly with the host or hostess of the party, you may be able to ascertain what they're serving at the party and know whether you can indulge in items at the gathering. Especially as we get older, we realize that more and more people have dietary restrictions. It is not uncommon for people to have restrictions and for hosts of parties to prepare for the restrictions of others. In society today, there are many people who are gluten-free, carb-free or have other food allergies. As a result, people are accustomed to preparing foods or having food available that people with such restrictions may eat while at the gatherings. So if you have a relationship with the host, you may be able to determine what they're serving and if you can bring something that suits your dietary needs as well as that of others.

If you are not in a position to be able to ask what is being served, and you don't feel comfortable bringing something of your own, it's a good idea to eat prior to leaving the house. That way, you will not feel like you must indulge due to hunger and you will be in a better frame of mind to pick and choose from the food offered. There is usually something that you will be able to eat at a party, even if it is not fulfilling. If you have eaten prior to leaving that you're home, you will not be ravenous and you can partake in the items that you are able to eat and leave the items that are not on your diet on the platter. If these gatherings involve alcohol, the keto diet only allows for the consumption of dry wines and hard spirits. If you are drinking hard liquor, use water or club soda as a mixer. Tonic water has carbohydrates in it and is not appropriate on the keto diet.

Keto at Restaurants

Eating in restaurants is not as difficult as eating in someone's home. Because of the sustained and massive interest in the ketogenic diet and other diets of its kind, there are many restaurants that offer low-carbohydrate versions of meals. At fast-food restaurants, typically you would simply order a burger or grilled chicken without the bun without ketchup or barbeque sauce Use lettuce as your bun. Of course, you will pass on the fries and onion rings. In general, fast food dining will not be your best option for eating out on a keto diet.

Restaurants with more items available, like sit-down restaurants, have larger menus and the choices often include many items that you can order or have modified and follow the ketogenic plan. The biggest problem you will have at these restaurants is the portion size. You need to be aware that the huge portion sizes are not going to be conducive to your eating plan. Remember to stay within your calories for the day. If you order food at a restaurant you will typically get enough food for two people. For this reason, you may want to split an entree with someone else who is dining with you. Also, if there are items on the menu with your entree that are not on the keto diet, request to have them left off your plate. This will save the kitchen waste and save you the temptation of eating items that are not on your diet plan. Many restaurants have their menu on the internet. It is a good idea to review the selections and have an idea of what you want to order when you get to the restaurant. Order two vegetables for sides of the entrees. Make sure the vegetables are ketogenic friendly. Stay away from the potatoes and the rice. You can generally order two vegetables. If you're not able to order to split an order, make sure you divide your order in half before you begin eating. Some people like to order the carryout container to be delivered with their food. This way they move half of their portion into the container before they start to eat. This is a good idea if you feel like you will not be able to stop eating once you start.

The keto diet is easy to follow in most restaurants in situations, but the portions are large and you should make sure you do not overeat and do not exceed your calorie counts nor other macros for in your restaurant meal.

Chapter 4: What are the Best Fats on Keto?

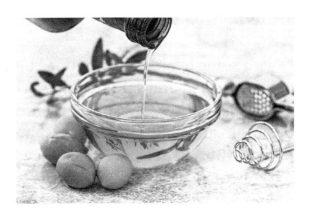

Fats are the most important part of the keto diet, but which fats are best for the diet? There are a variety of fats that can be used. The fat eaten on the keto diet makes up 70% of the food that you'll be eating each day. This makes the types of fats eaten important because all fats are not going to produce healthy weight loss on the keto diet. There are fats to be consumed and fats to be avoided. Just because fat is the predominant macro does that mean that consumption of unlimited fat is part of the keto diet. Stay within your calorie allotment for the day and watch your macros. Do not exceed your macros when you're eating fats. Most importantly, consume the correct types of fat to maximize the effectiveness of your fat intake.

Types of Fat
There are several types of fat and some are better than

others when it comes to overall health and usefulness as fuel for the body. Combine various types of fats that have proved to be the best fuel for the body.

Polyunsaturated Fatty Acids (PUFA)

These are fats with some health contributions but not as many as other unsaturated and saturated fats. This is the category where omega-3 fatty acids fall. Omega-3 fatty acids are good for the brain and should be included in a healthy diet. The problems with PFUAs arise when they are heated because they may, with heat, form compounds that cause inflammation, and I may damage the pancreas and liver.

Polyunsaturated fatty acids (PFUA) should be eaten cold to avoid the unstable reactions of PUFAs when heated. Some good PFUAs for the keto diet are extra virgin olive oil, nuts, avocados and avocado oil, and fatty fish.

Monounsaturated Fatty Acids (MUFAs)

These fats are the healthiest of unsaturated fats. They remain stable when heated and have a positive effect on insulin production and cholesterol levels. MUFAs assist the pancreas in producing and consistent levels of insulin. They are also known to reduce bad cholesterol levels (LDL) and improve overall blood pressure and heart health.

The MUFAs are commonly found in lard, bacon, macadamia nuts, sesame oil, and butter. These fats remain stable at higher temperatures and therefore have predictable reactions to heat. These oils can be moderately included in the keto diet.

Saturated Fats

These are the best fats for keto. They are found in animals, and other high-fat foods and are not the result of chemical processing. When eating fats on keto, hunger is assuaged by the consumption of saturated fats. These fats have a positive influence on the health of the body. Included in saturated fats is MCT oil. MCT stands for Medium Chain Triglycerides. The shorter length of triglyceride makes MCTs easier to digest and break down in the system. MCTs are known to improve brain function and reduce the growth of yeast and bacteria in the body. It's a beneficial oil while on keto.

Saturated fats are known to increase the amount of good cholesterol, HDL while decreasing the bad cholesterol, LDL. There is also an improvement to the immune system and an increase in bone density when saturated fats are present in the human body. This is a good side effect for women over 50 who may be suffering from bone loss.

Common foods that are good sources of healthy saturated fats are fatty meats like steak, butter and ghee, eggs, coconut oil, lard, and palm kernel oil. These items should be included in the majority of fat on the keto diet. Since the diet relies on the consumption of so much fat, there will be a need to eat a lot of these fats. This will be the healthiest way to provide fat as fuel for your body as you reduce the number of carbs in your diet.

Omega-3, Omega-6, Omega-9

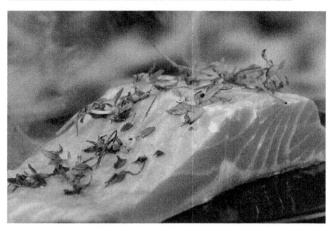

Omega-3 fatty acids are polyunsaturated fats that increase HDL and improve heart health. They decrease the fat in the liver and improve liver function. These fats also reduce the inflammation in your body and organs. Omega-3 fatty acids are key in reducing waist size and promoting weight loss. Foods high in omega-3 fatty acids are fish, like salmon, mackerel, and sardines. Walnuts and chia seeds are also high in Omega-3.

Omega-6 fatty acids are polyunsaturated fats that are used for energy. The problem is, most normal diets contain too much Omega-6. In large concentrations, the omega-6 fatty acids increase inflammation in the body and cause associated diseases like asthma, rheumatoid arthritis, ulcerative colitis, and sinusitis. Omega-6 fatty acids must be consumed in moderation so that negative effects do not overwhelm the positive. Some of the foods high in omega-6 are soybean oil, corn oil, mayonnaise, walnuts, and almonds. Eating these foods in moderation will be the best way to receive the benefits of omega-6 fatty acids.

Omega-9 fatty acids are monounsaturated fats that are found naturally in the body but may be consumed as well. These fats are found to improve the worst types of cholesterol in the body, reduce inflammation and improve insulin sensitivity. They may also improve metabolism when monounsaturated fats with omega-9 are consumed instead of saturated fats. Foods high in omega-9 are nut and seed oils like cashew oil, flaxseed oil, peanut oil, and olive oil. It is also found in olives as well as almonds, cashews, and walnuts. Moderate consumption of omega-9 fatty acids is appropriate because it is a natural part of the body's composition and tolerated well when introduced as food.

Fats play an important role in the keto diet. Foods with Omega-3 fatty acids should get added to your food plan two or three times a week. Omega-6 fatty acids should not be included in a grand way in the diet as they do not have as many positive effects on the body. Overconsumption of omega-6 can have negative effects on overall health. Omega-9 fatty acids are already found in the body so it isn't necessary to work hard getting it into your system.

*_Fat Bombs_*

With all the talk about fats, let's not overlook fat bombs. Fat bombs are high-fat morsels of food used to boost fat levels while on the keto diet. This is good if you find that you are not eating enough fat or feel hungry or lacking in energy. These items are high in fat, low in carbohydrates and combined into a small portion designed to boost energy, reduces cravings and fill you up so you don't feel hungry. Because of the small size, do not overindulge. They are meant to be small bites that last. Pay attention to your macros, even while indulging in little bursts of food energy.

Chapter 5: Negative Moments in Keto

Keto Flu

Keto flu is the feeling of fatigue, headache, and the lack of concentration similar to being sick with the flu. It occurs when eliminating carbohydrates from the system. The body is adjusting to the lack of carbohydrates by offering a barrage of warnings that something is missing. Eventually, the transition will be complete and energy will be derived from fat instead of carbohydrates, but how to get through the keto flu?

If possible, avoid the keto flu. To do this, gradually reduce the carbohydrates and your system, so your body is able to adapt from the primary energy source of carbohydrates to the new source of fat. Eliminate processed carbohydrates from your diet first. These carbohydrates are sugar, cereals, baked goods, and packaged items with preservatives and salt. Eliminating these foods will give a good start to avoiding the keto flu. It is good to kick off your quest for ketosis by getting rid of it the least healthy foods first. Next, stop eating grains. For many people, this is a difficult category of food to stop eating. The carbohydrates in bread, rice, wheat flour, and pasta provide a lot of energy in a regular diet. People consider many of these carbohydrates to be comfort food. It is hard to give them up. Fortunately, your body can adjust to being without them. Finally, eliminate fruits and starchy vegetables. Weaning yourself off carbs is a way to reduce the effects of withdrawal on the body as the fuel stores of carbohydrates and glucose are used up and ketosis takes over and your body begins getting energy from fat.

When you are reducing the number of carbohydrates, be sure to drink a lot of water. The reduction of carbohydrates will, from the start, release the water stored in your body and increase the frequency of urination. When you stay hydrated, that removes an unnecessary stressor from your system as you adjust to the reduction of carbohydrates. Also, replace electrolytes being removed with your frequent trips to the bathroom. Replenish them with high potassium, low carbohydrate foods like salmon, nuts, mushrooms, and green leafy vegetables. Trying to keep electrolytes in balance and avoid the keto flu. You may also supplement your hydration with bone broth. Heat the bone broth and add salt and seasonings this will help restore your electrolyte balance as well.

If you're unable to avoid the keto flu, you want to feel better fast. One of the best ways to manage the effects of keto flu is to drink lots of water and get lots of sleep. These two things reduce the amount of stress your body is feeling and allowed to switch the generation energy from carbohydrates def bad which will mean you're finally in ketosis. Stay the course and stick to the diet. The keto flu symptoms will eventually pass. If you and the bone broth to your diet while you're feeling the effects of the keto flu, it will provide essential nutrients and comfort from the warm of the beverage in your stomach. iI essence, you are treating the keto flu in the same way you would treat regular flu. Allow your body to rest and drink lots of water but stay the course on your diet so that you reach ketosis which will end your keto flu.

Constipation

You may find that as you eliminate grains from your diet, your bowel movements are not your friend. Your body should be able to adjust to the change in food over time but you may need to introduce foods that will promote easy evacuation. Doctors have said that difficulty in bowel movements is uncomfortable but not usually a serious ailment. You will probably be able to last for some time with the mental challenge of straining to poop, but you don't really want to endure the pain, so make sure you incorporate whole fiber whole grains into your diet so that you are able to move your bowels. Some suggestions are to add chia seeds and flax seeds to your diet in order to lessen the effects of constipation. Add chia seeds to water, stir and drink. The chia seeds don't have any flavor and even the pickiest eaters should be able to stomach the watery concoction. One or two tablespoons of chia seeds may be just what you need to relieve yourself of constipation. If you add the chia seeds to yogurt or smoothies, you run the risk of exceeding your carbohydrate macros. The problem with this yogurt and dairy tends to be high in carbohydrates so you may end up using your daily allotment of carbohydrates on one food item.

Diarrhea

On the other side of constipation is diarrhea. If you're

experiencing diarrhea on the keto diet, it may be as simple as your consuming too much fat and too much protein. When the fat and protein are not digested easily, they're not absorbed into your system and remain unused and diarrhea is the result. Consume more fiber and look at the fat you're eating. If you are not meeting your macros, make an effort to fix them. Try changing over to monounsaturated fats and MCTs that are easily absorbed into the body and that may be able to fix your problem with diarrhea. Brussel sprouts, avocado, and broccoli are keto-friendly soluble fibers that will help with constipation.

Dietary changes may upset your system and may show itself in a negative way through constipation or diarrhea and upset stomach. It's good to make notes of what you are eating and compare it to your macros to be sure that your every sure you're eating good fat and that some of your protein comes from some of your protein is coming from vegetable green leafy vegetables. Adding a whole grain may help, as well.

Insomnia

An inability to sleep may accompany your keto diet. Energy from carbohydrates is not sustained over long periods of time. As the carbohydrates are leaving the body, it may be that the body is not dependent on carbohydrates and does not experience the crash when the carbs are used up. It is usually a temporary condition,

To combat sleeplessness, try a few different things:

1. Eat your carbohydrates closer to bedtime. This may trick your body into a state of low energy in a simulation of what often happens when you get your energy from carbohydrates. Just as you have a burst of energy upon eating carbs, the energy is quickly dissipated, and a feeling of tiredness and lethargy ensues.
2. Replenish electrolytes in your body through potassium-rich foods that will provide essential nutrients to your body, which may be missing and through your body out of balance. Avocados, pumpkin seeds, and salmon are helpful foods in counteracting the loss of minerals.
3. Prepare for bed. Make sure the room is dark and comfortable, and consider meditation or yoga before bedtime.

<u>Diet Plateaus</u>

When you have been losing weight, and it suddenly stops, it can be an irritating situation. Plateaus are common in all diets. The body adjusts to what you are eating and what you are doing for exercise and settles in. To get through the plateau, a change will need to be made.

The first thing to do if your weight loss is slower than expected is to review your macros. Every four or five weeks, you should recalculate your macros to make adjustments for your weight loss. A plateau may be the result of overeating your macros. Be sure you are not exceeding your overall daily calorie count. If your calories are not all burned off with activity, you will not lose weight. Your calories expended must exceed calories eaten to lose weight. Keep track of everything you eat, even little things, and include them in your macros. It will help you know you are not exceeding overall calories.

If you are not exercising, exercise. If you are exercising, you may need to change your routine. Increased exercise will jolt the body into a new use of energy and be forced to burn more energy, and as a result, more fat. It isn't about where you are exercising or that you are in the gym or jogging; you may just need to add steps to your day or increase your activity. You just need to increase your movement.

If your macros are still accurate and you are not losing weight, consider measuring yourself on a regular basis, especially if you have added exercise and weight training to our daily routine. Muscle weighs more than fat, be sure you are not replacing fat with muscle. That is not a bad situation to be in, but you should know if you are actually doing well, and your body is gaining strength and muscle. If you have not adjusted your workout routine, this probably isn't the problem.

Other things that may cause weight gain are stress and sleeplessness, which causes stress in the body. Stress is something that causes the body to retain weight as it gears up to fight whatever it is that is causing the turmoil in your body. Exercise may help to relieve stress. So will meditation or yoga. The key is to relieve yourself of the stress so your body may be more efficiently working on your weight loss.

Cholesterol and Keto

There are many food staples of the keto diet that are known to increase cholesterol levels in humans. This is one of the reasons food quality is part of the diet plan. For some of the food items on the plan, the higher quality items have fewer negative effects on healthy eating.

Cholesterol is a type of fat in your blood. It is formed in the liver and distributed throughout the body through the arteries and veins. Cholesterol, in normal amounts, travels to the brain and helps the brain function and memory. It also helps in the generation of hormones and normal organ functions, including the largest organ, skin. If there is too much cholesterol in the blood, the fats cling to the walls of the veins and arteries and may cause clogs or restrict the flow of blood. When there is not enough blood moving to the heart, a heart attack may result. If there is not enough blood reaching the brain, a stroke may occur. This is why the level of cholesterol in the system is a key factor in determining the health of an individual.

Cholesterol is made up of two types of lipoprotein. There is low-density lipoprotein (LDL), which moves through the blood with the assistance of proteins and other substances in the blood that causes plaque. Plaque is what attaches the fat to the walls of the veins. This is why LDL is considered to be bad cholesterol. High-density lipoprotein (HDL) is healthy cholesterol. It does not accumulate as it moves through the bloodstream. It carries cholesterol with it as it moves through blood vessels and takes it to the liver where it is processed for evacuation from the body.

Since the keto diet is one that concentrates on consuming so much fat, choosing appropriate fats will give you some control over the type of cholesterol in your body. The body needs cholesterol to function properly, so the goal is to consume food products prone to add more HDL and minimal amounts of LDL to your blood. To do this, the fats you eat should not have trans fats. Trans fats are high in LDL. They are often found in packaged foods, fried foods, margarine, baked goods, and crackers. Well, most of these items are not part of the keto diet. When prepared with partially or hydrogenated cooking oils, even fried meats are subject to higher levels of LDL. They are often used because they are more stable at higher temperatures.

If you are eating the right fats and find that your cholesterol levels are being negatively affected by the keto diet, try changing what you are eating as well as the combinations of food. If you are following the gentle keto 10% carb diet try reducing the number of carbs in your diet. Studies have found that people on a low-carb diet have increased HDL levels while they are losing weight. You may also try to limit your oils consumed to extra virgin olive oil which has been found to increase HDL as it is less processed than some other oils. Increased exercise is a way to combat low levels of HDL. Exercise will help you lose more weight as well. Losing weight helps with cholesterol levels.

For most people, the keto diet will not adversely affect cholesterol levels and, in fact, may improve the ratios between HDL and LDL levels. If you have cholesterol concerns, check with your doctor to be sure it is monitored regularly. Each body is different, and so you may have to try different methods of controlling your cholesterol levels. With the help of your physician, you should be able to determine if changes are working. A lower weight may be the best improvement to your health.

Chapter 6: Keto Recipes

Breakfast

Keto-Friendly Breakfast Tortilla

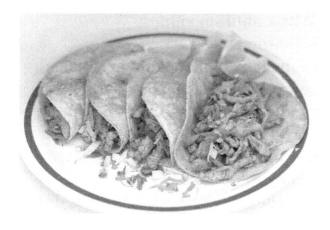

This breakfast tortilla recipe is replacing a flour burrito with an eggy wrap. This can be used to make an easy hand-held breakfast omelet for a compact keto breakfast.

Prep & Cooking Time: 10 mins

Servings: 1 tortilla
Nutrition Facts: Calories: 331 | Carbohydrates: 1g | Protein: 11g | Fat: 30g
Ingredients

1 T. butter
2 large eggs
2 T cream cheese
1 t. chilli powder
salt to taste

Instructions:

1. Melt cream cheese in a microwave for 10 seconds at a time until soft. Whisk until smooth.
2. Mix in eggs, chili powder, and salt.
3. Melt butter in a pan on medium heat. When melted, pour egg mixture in a pan and spread around in a circle. To thinly and evenly coat the bottom of the pan.
4. Turn the heat to low and cover the pan, so the top of the egg mixture cooks.
5. Leave on heat until the top of the egg mixture is dry- around 2 minutes.
6. Slide out egg onto the pan onto a plate.
7. Fill the keto tortilla with your choice of meat, cheese, and vegetables.
8. Roll up the "tortilla" and eat immediately or let cool and wrap in paper to enjoy later.

Breakfast Sandwich

You don't need bread when you can use sausage instead. The sausage patties are easy to handle and prove the perfect accompaniment to the eggs and cheese for with plenty of fat to start your keto day. This is perfect as a 'breakfast for dinner' meal if you add a vegetable like spinach or baby kale instead of avocado.

Prep & Cooking Time: 15 mins

Servings: 1 sandwich
Nutrition Facts: Calories: 603 | Carbohydrates: 7g | Protein: 22g | Fat: 54g

Ingredients:

2 pork sausage patties
1 large egg
1 T cream cheese
2 T sharp cheddar or extra sharp cheddar cheese

¼ medium avocado, sliced

Sriracha to taste
Salt and pepper to taste

Instructions

1. Cook sausages in a skillet over medium heat until the sausage is cooked through. Do this according to the package instructions.
2. Place the cream cheese and cheddar cheese in a microwave-safe bowl. Heat the cheeses until melted. This will take 20 or 30 seconds depending on your microwave.
3. Add sriracha to the cheese to taste and set the bowl aside.
4. Beat eggs in a different bowl and add salt and pepper as desired.
5. Coat frying pan with oil and butter. Cook egg as omelet until done.
6. Add avocado to egg, fold, and remove from pan.
7. Spread both sausage patties with cream cheese mixture.
8. Assemble the sandwich by layering sausage, egg, and top with a sausage patty.
9. Serve while hot.

Banana Nut Muffins

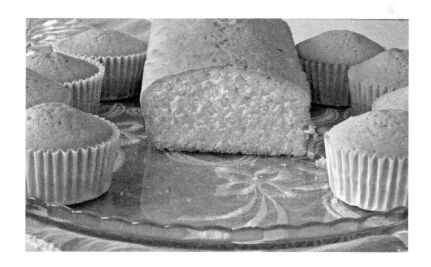

That's right; banana muffins are keto. Just use banana extract instead of bananas to get that familiar flavor. The muffin makes a great nut-holder as well. This is keto baking at its finest.

Prep & Cooking Time: 45 mins

Servings: 1 muffin
Nutrition Facts: Calories: 184 | Carbohydrates: 7g | Protein: 7g | Fat: 14g

Ingredients:

1 ¼ c almond flour
¼ c stevia
2 t baking powder

½ t ground cinnamon
⅓ c butter, melted
2 ½ t banana extract
¼ c unsweetened vanilla almond milk

¼ c sour cream
2 large eggs, slightly beaten
¾ c finely chopped walnuts or pecans

Topping:

1 T cold butter cut into pieces

1 T almond flour
½ T stevia

Instructions:

Preheat oven to 350 degrees
Grease a muffin tin with butter or line with 10 muffin liners.

Mix muffins

1. In a large bowl, mix dry ingredients, including the cinnamon.
2. Stir in melted butter, banana extract, almond milk, and sour cream.
3. Add eggs and nuts to the mixture and mix until all ingredients are incorporated.
4. Fill muffin cups with batter to half full.

Crumble topping:
1. Pulse the cold butter, almond flour, and stevia in a food processor until crumbly. If the mixture appears too dry, add another tablespoon of butter to pulse a few more times.
2. Sprinkle topping on top of muffins evenly.

Bake: 20 minutes.

Remove from oven when golden brown and they appear cooked. Let cool before eating. The texture will not be the same as a muffin but denser. They are still tasty little bites for breakfast.

Smoothies and Beverages

Coconut Green Smoothie

This smoothie has coconut oil and coconut milk as a wonderful pick-me-up when you need a shot of fiber. Enjoy the fresh coconut flavor that is balanced with matcha. It is a refreshing drink for any time.

Prep Time: 5 mins

Servings: 1 smoothie
Nutrition Facts: Calories: 341 | Carbohydrates: 3.9g | Protein: 5.6g | Fat: 24.7g

Ingredients:
⅔ c slightly defrosted frozen chopped spinach
½ avocado
1 T coconut oil
½ t matcha powder
1 T monk fruit sweetener
½ c coconut milk (from the dairy section, not canned)
⅔ c water
½ cup of ice

Instructions:

1. Add all ingredients except the ice into a blender. Blend until everything is blended well.

2. Pulse in the ice until it is evenly distributed.
3. Pour into a glass.

This smoothie is good for fiber and fat. You can add flaxseed or softened chia seeds to the smoothie for additional fiber and nutrients. Fresh spinach can be used and may be substituted with fresh or frozen kale.

Strawberry Smoothie

Add a touch of sweetness to your day with this strawberry smoothie. This smoothie is good enough for dessert. If you want to add some fiber and protein, try adding chia seeds that have been softened in water. 2 tablespoons of chia will add 139 calories, 1 gram of carbohydrate, 4 grams of protein, and 9 grams of fat.

Prep Time: 5 mins

Servings: 1 smoothie
Nutrition Facts: Calories: 302 | Carbohydrates: 8g | Protein: 2g | Fat: 26g

Ingredients:

¼ c heavy cream
¾ c unsweetened vanilla almond milk
2 t stevia
½ c frozen strawberries (whole or sliced)

½ c ice (preferably crushed)

Instructions:

1. Blend ingredients in a blender until blended well.
2. Pour into a tall glass.
3. Serve.

Keto Mojito

Yes! There are keto-friendly cocktails. It takes a little preparation; stevia is used instead of sugar, but you don't need a blender. Muddling the mint leaves releases the mint fragrance and provides the minty backdrop for this refreshing drink. This is an easy recipe that is festive and interactive (muddling) for a fun part beverage.

Prep Time: 4 mins

Servings: 1 mojito
Nutrition Facts: Calories: 109 | Carbohydrates: 2g

Ingredients
4 fresh mint leaves
2 T fresh lime Juice
2 t stevia
Ice

1.5 oz shot of white rum
splash club soda or plain seltzer
fresh mint as garnish

Instructions:

1. Muddle the mint, lime juice, and stevia for 10 seconds in the glass in which the drink will be served.
2. Fill the glass with ice, either cubed or crushed.
3. Pour the shot of vodka over the ice.
4. Add club soda to fill the glass
5. Garnish with a mint leaf.

You may want to strain the drink after muddling to remove the broken mint leaves, so they don't get in the way of enjoying the drink. You can substitute vodka or gin for rum.

Soup

Chicken and Riced Cauliflower Soup

To make this soup keto-friendly, riced cauliflower is used to add that missing texture to the soup. It is a hearty soup that will remind you of homemade soups from home...or the deli. It makes a nice lunch or snack. Make a batch on the weekend and take it for lunch through the week.

Prep & Cooking Time: 40 mins

Servings: 4 Servings
Nutrition Facts: Calories: 196 | Carbohydrates: 4.8g | Protein: 26.4g | Fat: 10.4g

Ingredients:

2 T olive oil
2 stalks celery with tops, chopped
¼ c onions, chopped
salt and pepper, to taste
2 cloves garlic, minced
½ t paprika
4 c unsalted organic chicken bone broth
2 c chicken thigh meat, cut into 1/2" cubes
2 c riced cauliflower

Instructions:

1. Heat the oil in a large saucepan over medium heat.
2. Add celery and onions and season with salt and pepper. Cook, stirring frequently, until vegetables are tender, about 5 minutes.
3. Add garlic and paprika. If needed, add another tablespoon of olive oil to the pan with the garlic, so the garlic cooks evenly. Saute and cook until garlic is soft. This will take a minute or so.
4. Stir in chicken bone broth and bring to a boil.
5. Add chicken and riced cauliflower and simmer the soup until the chicken is cooked and the cauliflower is tender, but not overcooked.
6. Season with additional salt and pepper to taste.
7. Serve hot.

Spicy Creamy Chicken Soup

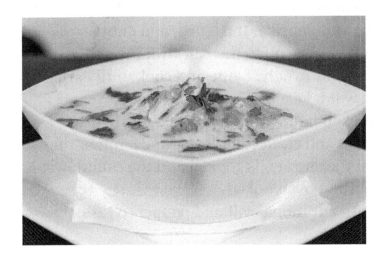

This recipe uses a slow-cooker to make soup in one pot. It is a spicy soup that has a lot of flavors and is high in fat. The heat of the jalapeño is offset by the cream cheeses. The soup tastes like a taco dip with chicken. Use the bone in chicken breasts to keep the chicken from drying out for the slow cook on low heat.

Prep & Cooking Time: 4 hrs 20 mins

Servings: 4 Servings
Nutrition Facts: Calories: 424 | Carbohydrates: 6g | Protein: 41g | Fat: 25g

Ingredients:

1 lb chicken breasts on the bone
1 c onion, diced
4 cloves garlic, minced
1 jalapeño pepper, chopped
1 T cumin
½ T chili powder
1 t salt
3 T lime juice
2 c low sodium organic chicken broth
1 8 oz package of cream cheese
½ c cilantro, chopped

Instructions:

1. Add the chicken, onion, garlic, jalapeño, cumin, chili powder, paprika, salt, lime juice, and chicken broth to a slow cooker.
2. Cook in the slow-cooker, covered, for 4 hours on the lowest setting.
3. After chicken is cooked through, remove from the pot and let cool until it can be easily handled.
4. Pull the chicken off the bone and shred or chop into bite-sized pieces.
5. Add the cream cheese to hot soup. Stir slowly until melted.
6. Add shredded chicken into the pot and stir to mix.
7. Bring the soup back up to temperature and turn off the heat.
8. Spoon into bowls and sprinkle cilantro on top.

9. Serve immediately.

Add a sprinkle of cheddar to add cheesy flavor to the soup.

Broccoli Cheese Soup

This is a thick and hearty soup that only has 5 ingredients. This can serve as a quick, last-minute meal that will please everyone. If you want to make it even more hearty, add tender cooked cubes of beef.

Prep & Cooking Time: 45 mins

Servings: 6 Servings
Nutrition Facts: Calories: 291 | Carbohydrates: 4g | Protein: 13g | Fat: 25g

Ingredients:

4 c broccoli florets
4 cloves minced garlic
3 ½ c low sodium vegetable broth
1 c heavy cream
3 c shredded sharp cheddar cheese

INSTRUCTIONS

1. In a large pot, sauté garlic in butter, ghee, or olive oil for one minute over medium heat.
2. Add vegetable broth, heavy cream, and chopped broccoli.
3. Heat soup to boiling, then reduce heat and simmer for 10-20 minutes, until broccoli is tender.
4. Use an immersion blender to puree the broccoli in the soup. If you do not have an immersion blender, use a slotted spoon to remove the broccoli and blend in a blender or food processor. After the broccoli is pureed, stir it back into the soup pot.
5. Reduce the heat under the soup and slowly add the cheddar into the soup, stirring frequently until melted.
6. Puree the soup again with the stick blender or regular blender.
7. Remove the soup from heat and serve in bowls.

Sauces and Dips

Tzatziki

Tzatziki can be used as a sauce or topping or dip. It is so versatile; add it to a salad of lettuce, tomato, olives, and arugula. It can be a dip for meat skewers or a spread for a keto-friendly sandwich. Tzatziki is a fresh, light addition to any snack or meal.

Prep Time: 10 mins

Servings: 8 Servings, 2 tablespoons per serving
Nutrition Facts: Calories: 79 | Carbohydrates: 3g | Protein: 1g | Fat: 7g

Ingredients:

½ c shredded cucumber, drained
1 tsp salt
1 T olive oil
1 T fresh mint, finely chopped
2 garlic cloves
1 c full-fat Greek yogurt
1 t lemon juice

Instructions:

1. Place shredded cucumber on a strainer for an hour or squeeze out moisture through a cheesecloth.
2. Mix all ingredients in a medium bowl
3. Refrigerate.

Use as a vegetable dip, a dip for dehydrated vegetables, or a sauce for lamb, beef, or chicken. It is also a perfect accompaniment for fried summer squash.

Satay Sauce

Bring a bit of Thailand into your kitchen with this satay sauce recipe. This is a great use for peanut butter and coconut cream. It is simply delicious and naturally keto-friendly.

Prep & Cooking Time: 15 mins

Servings: 4 Servings
Nutrition Facts: Calories: 312 | Carbohydrates: 7g | Protein: 7g | Fat: 30g

Ingredients:
1 can (14 oz) coconut cream (if you can't find coconut cream, coconut milk works well)
1 dry red pepper, seeds removed, chopped fine
1 clove garlic, minced
¼ c gluten-free soy sauce

⅓ c natural unsweetened peanut butter
salt and pepper

Instructions:

1. Place all ingredients in a small saucepan.
2. Bring the mixture to a boil
3. Stir while heating to mix peanut butter with other ingredients as it melts.
4. After the mixture boils, turn down the heat to simmer on low heat for 5 to 10 minutes.
5. Remove from heat when the sauce is at the desired consistency.
6. Adjust seasoning to taste.

This is a good sauce for chicken or turkey. Just add the sauce during the last minutes of baking or grilling. It can also be used as a dipping sauce.

Thousand Island Salad Dressing

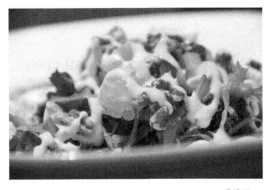

If you need a salad dressing, thousand island is popular on salads and as a sandwich spread. This adaptation makes the dressing keto-friendly for both purposes.

Prep & Cooking Time: 5 mins

Servings: 8 Servings
Nutrition Facts: Calories: 312 | Carbohydrates: 2g | Protein: 1g | Fat: 34g

Ingredients:

2 T olive oil
¼ c frozen spinach, thawed
2 T dried parsley
1 T dried dill
1 t onion powder
½ t salt
¼ t black pepper
1 c full-fat mayonnaise
¼ c full-fat sour cream
2 t lemon juice

Instructions:

1. Mix all ingredients in a small bowl.
2. Enjoy

This dressing can be covered and stored for up to 5 days.

Hollandaise Sauce

Since asparagus is a staple on keto diet plans, here is the traditional hollandaise sauce to accompany your spears. The sauce works on any vegetables. You will need to use a double-boiler for this sauce

Prep & Cooking Time: 25 mins

Servings: 4 Servings
Nutrition Facts: Calories: 566 | Carbohydrates: 1g | Protein: 3g | Fat: 62g

Ingredients:

4 egg yolks
2 T lemon juice
1 ½ sticks of butter, melted
salt and pepper

Instructions:

1. Heat water to boil in a saucepan.
2. Separate the eggs. Save the whites for another use.
3. Place the yolks in a heat-resistant bowl, either glass or stainless steel.
4. Carefully melt the butter in a saucepan without burning.

5. Place the bowl with the egg yolks over the simmering water to gently heat the eggs. Make sure the water is not touching the bottom of the bowl. The eggs need to be steamed, not cooked.
6. Add lemon juice to egg yolks.
7. Slowly stream the melted butter into the egg yolks while whisking. Start with a few drops of butter and then add a slow stream. Whisk the eggs the entire time until all the butter is added and the sauce has thickened.
8. Season to taste with lemon juice, salt, and pepper. You can also add a dash of tabasco sauce.
9. Serve over poached eggs or cooked vegetables.

Side Dishes

Mexican Cauliflower Rice

Give your cauliflower rice a spicy flair with this recipe. It's easy and quick and will be even faster using frozen cauliflower rice that has been thawed and drained in place of fresh.

Prep & Cooking Time: 25 mins

Servings: 8 Servings
Nutrition Facts: Calories: 90 | Carbohydrates: 4g | Protein: 3g | Fat: 8g

Ingredients:

1 head of cauliflower, riced
¼ c butter
⅓ c onion, minced
⅓ c tomatoes, diced
1 clove garlic, minced
¼ c jalapeño pepper, minced
1 T tomato paste
1 T chilli powder
½ t ground cumin
2 T lime juice
2 t olive oil
1 t salt

3 T fresh cilantro, chopped
¼ cup sharp cheddar cheese, optional

Instruction:

1. Wash cauliflower and grate to a texture resembling rice. This can also be done in a food processor. Set aside.
2. In a large skillet, heat pan to medium heat and melt butter. Sauté onion and garlic in the butter until soft.
3. Add tomatoes, jalapeño pepper, tomato paste, olive oil, chili powder, and cumin and stir until well mixed.
4. When the mixture in the pan is soft and fragrant, add riced cauliflower, lime juice, and salt.
5. Cook until riced cauliflower is the texture you prefer.
6. Top with fresh cilantro and cheddar cheese.
7. Serve while hot.

Green Beans and Bacon

This is a nice holiday side dish, but it can be a decadent dish for a regular day. It is fast and easy but tastes like it took hours to prepare. Combining bacon and a vegetable is also a good way to get non-vegetable eaters to give the green bean a try.

Prep & Cooking Time: 30 mins

Servings: 4 Servings
Nutrition Facts: Calories: 235 | Carbohydrates: 6g | Protein: 6g | Fat: 19g

Ingredients:

1 lb fresh green beans cut to 1" pieces
½ t salt
6 cloves garlic, minced
6 strips of raw bacon, chopped to ½ inch pieces

Instructions:

1. Boil green beans in water and salt to al dente. This should take about ten minutes.
2. Drain beans after they reach the desired texture and set aside.
3. In a large skillet, cook bacon until pieces are crisp.

4. Drain off all but 2 tablespoons of the bacon fat.
5. Add green beans into the pan with the bacon pieces and bacon fat.
6. Continue cooking green beans in bacon fat another 3 to 4 minutes until soft.
7. Add garlic and season with salt to taste.
8. Serve hot.

Baked Spaghetti Squash

Like pasta, but no pasta carbs. This can be a side dish that satisfies your carb cravings. Serve it as a side dish or add a protein and top with cheese to make it an entree.

Prep & Cooking Time: 45 mins

Servings: 4 Servings
Nutrition Facts: Calories: 31 | Carbohydrates: 7g | Protein: .6g | Fat: .6g

Ingredients:

1 spaghetti squash
1 T olive oil
1 t sea salt
1 t pepper

Instructions:

1. Preheat oven to 400 degrees.
2. Cut spaghetti squash in half lengthwise.
3. Set squash on cooking pan, cut side up.
4. Sprinkle olive oil, salt, and pepper over the squash halves.
5. Bake for 40 minutes until soft.
6. Remove squash from the oven and allow it to cool until it is easy to handle.
7. Scrape the squash out of the shell into a bowl.
8. Season with additional salt and pepper to taste.

This dish is easy to prepare and satisfying.

Snacks

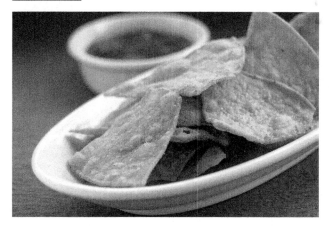

Taco Flavored Cheddar Crisps

Prep & Cooking Time: 15 mins

Servings: 6 Servings

Ingredients:

¾ c sharp cheddar cheese, finely shredded
¼ c parmesan cheese, finely shredded
¼ t chili powder
¼ t ground cumin

Instructions:

1. Preheat the oven to 400 degrees.
2. Line cookie sheet with parchment paper.

3. In a bowl, toss all ingredients together until well mixed.
4. Make 12 piles of cheese parchment paper.
5. Press down the cheese into a thin layer of cheese.
6. Bake for 5 minutes until cheese if bubby.
7. Allow to cool on parchment paper.
8. When completely cool, peel the paper away from the crisps.

These are a good keto substitute for chips. They are cheesy and crisp. Enjoy!

Keto Seed Crispy Crackers

With crackers being a pre-keto snack of the past, it is nice to be able to make a crispy cracker that can be served with cheese or spread with butter.

Prep & Cooking Time: 55 mins

Servings: 30 Servings of 1 cracker
Nutrition Facts: Calories: 61 | Carbohydrates: 1g | Protein: .2g | Fat: .6g

Ingredients:

1/3 cup almond flour
1/3 cup sunflower seed kernels
1/3 cup pumpkin seed kernels
1/3 cup flaxseed
1/3 cup chia seeds
1 tbsp ground psyllium husk powder
1 tsp salt
1/4 cup melted coconut oil
1 cup boiling water

Instructions:

1. Preheat the oven to 300 degrees.

2. Stir all dry ingredients together in a medium-sized bowl until thoroughly mixed.
3. Add coconut oil and boiling water to dry ingredients and stir until all ingredients are mixed well.
4. On a flat surface, roll the dough between two pieces of parchment paper until approximately ⅛ inch thick.
5. Slide the dough, still between parchment paper onto a baking sheet.
6. Remove the top layer of parchment paper and place dough on a baking sheet into the oven.
7. Bake 40 minutes until golden brown.
8. Score the top of the dough into cracker sized pieces.
9. Leave in the oven to cool down.
10. When the big cracker is cool, break into pieces.

These crackers can be stored in an airtight container after they are completely cool.

Beef – Pork – Chicken

Slow Cooker Chilli

This chili is very tasty. The meat can be prepared ahead of time and transferred to the slow cooker when it's time to start cooking. Including celery gives the chili the texture missing without beans.

Prep & Cooking Time: 6 hrs 15 mins

Servings: 6 Servings
Nutrition Facts: Calories: 137 | Carbohydrates: 4.7g | Protein: 16g| Fat: 5g

Ingredients:

2 ½ lbs ground beef
1 red onion, diced
5 cloves garlic, minced
1 ½ c celery, diced
1 6-ounce can tomato paste
1 14.5 oz can diced tomatoes with green chilies

1 14.5 oz can stewed tomatoes
4 T chili powder
2 T ground cumin
2 t salt
1 t garlic powder

1 t onion powder

3 t cayenne pepper

1 t red pepper flakes

Instructions:

1. Cook ground beef in a large skillet.
2. Add onion, garlic, and celery and cook until ground beef browned
3. Drain the fat from the beef
4. Place beef and vegetable mixture into the slow cooker set on a low setting.
5. Add tomatoes and seasonings then stir to mix.
6. Place the lid on the slow cooker and cook on low for 6 hours.

Serve with cheese on top if desired. Adjust the red pepper to taste.

Chicken Parmesan

Chicken, sauce, and cheese make this low carb chicken dish delicious. It's easy to prepare so you can serve it even when you have a busy day. For a slightly less traditional, higher-fat version, use chicken thighs or boneless, skinless pork chops.

Prep & Cooking Time: 40 mins

Servings: 4 Servings
Nutrition Facts: Calories: 309 | Carbohydrates: 9g | Protein: 37g| Fat: 4g

Ingredients:

2 ¼ lb boneless skinless chicken breasts

1 T Italian seasoning
½ t onion powder
½ t salt
1 T olive oil
¼ c onion, chopped
4 cloves garlic, minced
1 bell pepper, diced
1 28 oz can crushed tomatoes
½ c shredded mozzarella
¼ c shredded parmesan

Instructions:

1. Preheat oven to 350 degrees.
2. Coat chicken breasts with Italian seasoning, onion powder, and salt
3. Heat skillet pan and add olive oil when hot.
4. Cook chicken, browning on each side until chicken is just done.
5. Remove chicken from pan and arrange in one layer in an oven-safe baking dish.
6. Using the same skillet as the chicken, cook onion, garlic, and bell pepper until soft.
7. Pour as much of can of tomatoes into the hot skillet as fits and stir until vegetables are incorporated into the tomatoes.
8. Pour any excess tomatoes over chicken, then pour the hot tomatoes sauce over the chicken.
9. Top with cheese.
10. Bake in preheated oven for 10-15 minutes until hot and bubbly and cheese is melted and golden brown.

If you need to sneak some low carb vegetables into the dish, add finely chopped raw spinach or broccoli into the sauce or sprinkle over the chicken before the sauce is poured.

Baked Un-BBQ Ribs

These ribs are proof you don't need a sugary sauce to enjoy ribs. The tangy flavor is from lime juice and lots of seasonings. You don't have to rely on packaged and bottled sauces and rubs to create a delicious pork centerpiece for your next meal.

Prep & Cooking Time: 1hrs 40 mins

Servings: 6 Servings
Nutrition Facts: Calories: 445 | Carbohydrates: 3g | Protein: 37g| Fat: 32g

Ingredients:

2 slabs baby back ribs
2 T olive oil
1 T garlic powder
1 t onion powder
1 t paprika
1 t salt
1 tsp cayenne pepper
Juice of 2 limes

Instructions:

1. Preheat oven to 350 degrees.
2. Remove membrane from the back of each slab of ribs.

3. Put remaining ingredients in a covered bottle or jar and shake well to mix.
4. Lay ribs on an aluminum foil-covered baking sheet, bone side down.
5. Pour seasonings over ribs, rubbing into the meat. Make sure both sides of both slabs get seasoning.
6. Reserve ¼ of the seasonings.
7. Flip ribs over every 30 minutes to brown both sides of the rib slabs.
8. About one hour into the cooking time, pour reserved seasonings over the top of the ribs.
9. Cook ribs until tender, should be about an hour and a half.

Season with salt and pepper as needed. This is a flavorful and enjoyable protein, worth saving your protein macros.

Fish

Salmon skewers

This recipe can be an appetizer or an entree. This is an easy, quick meal that is fun and interactive. We love to pick up our food and eat with our fingers. If prosciutto is unavailable, you can always use bacon.

Prep & Cooking Time: 30 mins

Servings: 4 Servings
Nutrition Facts: Calories: 680 | Carbohydrates: 1g | Protein: 28g| Fat: 62g

Ingredients:

¼ c fresh spinach, chopped fine
1 lb salmon cut into bite-sized pieces
¼ t black pepper, freshly ground
½ t pink Himalayan salt
1 T olive oil
3½ oz sliced prosciutto
1 c full-fat mayonnaise

8 wooden or metal skewers

Instructions:

1. Heat oven to 400 degrees.
2. Mix olive oil spinach salt and pepper in a 1-gallon storage bag.
3. Coat salmon pieces in oil mixture by placing them in the bag.
4. Place salmon on skewers.
5. Wrap salmon skewers with prosciutto.
6. Bake salmon for approximately 15 minutes turning every 3 or 4 minutes.
7. When prosciutto is crispy, and salmon is cooked, remove from oven.
8. Serve with mayonnaise on the side.

This dish is flavorful, and the prosciutto adds a smokiness to the salmon. Dress up the mayo with a teaspoon of garlic for extra zest.

Coconut Salmon with Napa Cabbage

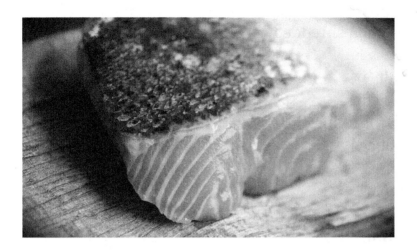

If you want to add an exotic flair to your salmon, try this recipe. The coconut and coconut oil give the dish a tropical feel. For a dipping sauce, try mixing Greek yogurt with turmeric and coconut cream. That will turn this delicious entree into finger food. Explore your exotic side with this salmon and Napa cabbage dish.

Prep & Cooking Time: 40 mins

Servings: 4 Servings
Nutrition Facts: Calories: 744 | Carbohydrates: 3g | Protein: 32g| Fat: 67g

Ingredients:

1¼ lbs salmon
1 T olive oil
½ c unsweetened shredded coconut
1 t turmeric
1 t kosher salt
½ t garlic powder
4 T olive oil, for frying
2 c Napa cabbage
1 stick butter
salt and pepper

Instructions:

1. Cut salmon into small 1-inch chunks.
2. Grind coconut to make it more likely to stay on the fish pieces. If you don't have a grinder, use a sharp knife to chop the shredded coconut as finely as possible.
3. Mix coconut, turmeric, salt, and garlic powder in a bowl.
4. In another bowl, coat salmon with 1 tablespoon of olive oil. Take
5. Dredge oil-coated salmon in dry ingredients.
6. Heat 4 tablespoons of olive oil in a frying pan to medium heat.
7. Cook coconut coated salmon until crispy. It will take about one minute per side. Make sure each side gets nicely browned.

8. Remove cooked salmon from the pan and keep warm while cooking the cabbage
9. Slice cabbage into thin strips with a knife or shred in a food processor.
10. Melt butter in pan used to cook salmon.
11. Cook cabbage until tender.
12. Season cabbage with salt and pepper.
13. Serve cabbage with salmon and enjoy.

Keto Tuna Casserole

If tuna casserole is one of your comfort dishes, this will be a keto version is a great way to satisfy tuna casserole needs. It is both economical and delicious, so a perfect fit if you are trying to do keto on a budget.

Prep & Cooking Time: 40 mins

Servings: 4 Servings
Nutrition Facts: Calories: 953 | Carbohydrates: 5g | Protein: 43g| Fat: 83g

Ingredients:

4 T butter
2 T olive oil
1 medium onion, diced
1 green bell pepper, diced

5 celery stalks, diced
2 c baby spinach chopped fine
2 large cans tuna in olive oil, drained
1 c mayonnaise
1 ½ c freshly shredded Parmesan cheese
1 t red pepper flakes
salt and pepper

Introduction:

1. Preheat oven to 350 degrees.
2. Heat butter and olive oil in a large skillet.
3. Sauté onions, green bell pepper, celery, and spinach in butter/oil.
4. In a bowl, mix tuna, Parmesan cheese, mayonnaise, and red pepper flake until thoroughly combined.
5. Add sautéed vegetables to the tuna mixture and stir until everything is incorporated
6. Pour tuna mixture into a casserole dish for baking.
7. Bake in the oven for 30 minutes.
8. Remove casserole from the oven when golden brown on top and bubbly.

This is a warm and comforting tuna dish that is quick to make. You can make the casserole the day before and store it in the refrigerator. Increase the baking time to 40 minutes when you put the cold casserole in the oven.

Vegetarian

Cinnamon Crunch Cereal

This is a vegetarian breakfast delight that is low in carbohydrates. It makes it easy to keep your protein macros in line when you need to eat less. This crispy sweet treat uses just a little stevia. You can adjust the sugar amount if necessary.

Prep & Cooking Time: 1 hr 40 mins

Servings: 6 Servings
Nutrition Facts: Calories: 129| Carbohydrates: 1g | Protein: 5g| Fat: 9g

Ingredients:

½ c flaxseed meal
½ c hemp seed meal
2 T ground cinnamon
½ t stevia
½ c water
1 T coconut oil

Instructions:

1. Preheat oven to 300 degrees.

2. Combine the dry ingredients (including stevia) in the bowl of a food processor.
3. Add water and coconut oil and mix until fully combined.
4. Add the apple juice and coconut oil and process until fully combined and mostly smooth.
5. Turn the batter onto a cookie sheet lined with parchment paper.
6. Spread it very thinly over the entire sheet.
7. Bake in the oven for 15 minutes.
8. After the 15 minutes are up, turn the heat down in the oven to 250 degrees.
9. Bake for an additional 5-7 minutes.
10. Remove the pan from the oven and cut the sheet of cereal into little squares. They should be small enough to fit on your spoon and eat.
11. Turn off the oven and put the cereal into the hot and cooling oven.
12. Leave in the oven for an hour,

This is a good cereal or snack. The recipe makes 6 ½ cup servings. It is so crunchy and delicious you will be tempted to snack throughout the day. This is good when you have used most of your macros but want a little something more.

Broccoli Cheese Fritters

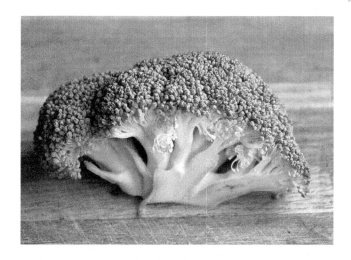

If you are a fan of corn fritters, these broccoli cheese fritters will be just what you are waiting for. Bursting with flavor, these morsels are

Prep & Cooking Time: 40 mins

Servings: 16 fritters w/sauce
Nutrition Facts: Calories: 104| Carbohydrates: 2g | Protein: 5g| Fat: 8g

Ingredients:

<u>Fritters</u>
¾ cup almond flour
7 T flaxseed meal
½ c fresh broccoli

½ c sharp cheddar cheese
2 large eggs
2 t baking powder
½ t hot sauce (without sugar)
Salt and Pepper to taste

Dipping Sauce
¼ c mayonnaise
¼ c cilantro, chopped
½ T lemon juice
Salt and pepper to taste

Instructions:

1. In a food processor, pulse broccoli until it is all in small uniform pieces.
2. In a separate bowl, mix almond flour, half of the flaxseed meal, and cheese.
3. Add eggs, hot sauce, and broccoli to the dry mixture and mix well.
4. Roll the batter into balls.
5. Put remaining flaxseed meal onto a plate.
6. Roll the batter ball in flaxseed meal to coat. Set on a plate or paper towel until fry time.
7. Heat up oil in a deep fat fryer to 375 degrees.
8. Put fritters on the basket and fry until brown. This will take from 3 to 5 minutes.
9. Fry in batches so there the basket is not crowded, and the fritters cook evenly.
10. Remove golden brown fritters from the fryer and drain on a rack with a paper towel underneath.

11. Season with salt and pepper.
12. Mix ingredients of dipping sauce in a bowl.

These fritters pair well with the dipping sauce. They are a nice keto-friendly addition to a meal or serve as snacks on game day. Finally, tailgating food that can be appreciated by everyone. They will not even realize the lack of cornmeal and white flour.

Asian Noodle Salad

This salad utilizes shirataki noodles, which are keto-friendly because they are mostly water. This makes a nice change while on a low-carb diet if you miss pasta. The Asian flavors are present in the salad and dressing. Eat it as an accompaniment to a meal or as an entire meal in itself. The flavor is fresh and delightful with all of the fresh vegetables, with Asian seasoning.

Prep & Cooking Time: 30 mins

Servings: 4 servings
Nutrition Facts: Calories: 212 | Carbohydrates: 6g | Protein: 7g| Fat: 16g

Ingredients:

<u>Salad</u>
1 c shredded red cabbage

1 c shredded green cabbage
¼ c scallions, chopped
⅓ c cilantro, chopped
4 c shirataki noodles, prepared and drained
¼ c chopped peanuts

Dressing
2 T garlic, minced
½ c water
1 T lime juice
1 T sesame oil
1 T gluten-free soy sauce
¼ c natural, unsweetened peanut butter
¼ t cayenne pepper
½ t salt
½ t stevia

Instructions:

1. Mix salad ingredients in a large bowl.
2. Place dressing ingredients in a blender and blend until smooth.
3. Pour dressing over salad and toss to coat salad with dressing completely.

This can be served room temperature or cold as a side dish or entree. Refrigerate any unused salad in an airtight container.

Dessert

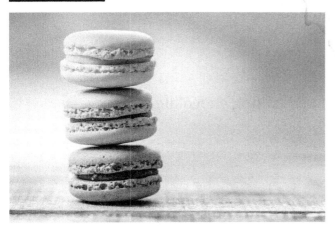

Cocoa Brownies

Like conventional brownies, all you need are the ingredients, and you can have brownies in an hour. The chocolate flavor comes through because there is so much of it. The sweetener tastes natural and a nearly flourless chocolate confection is created with only a few carbs. Thanks to the use of butter, the fat grams per browning are abundant.

Prep & Cooking Time: 40 mins

Servings: 9 servings
Nutrition Facts: Calories: 201 | Carbohydrates: 5g | Protein: 3g | Fat: 19g

Ingredients:

½ c salted butter, melted
1 c Granular Swerve Sweetener
2 Large Eggs
2 t vanilla extract
12 squares unsweetened baking chocolate, melted

2 T coconut flour
2 T cocoa powder
½ T baking powder
½ t salt
½ c walnuts, chopped (optional)

Instructions:

1. Preheat oven to 350 degrees.
2. Spray square baking pan with cooking spray or grease pan well with butter.
3. In a large mixing bowl, use an electric mixer or whisk and mix together butter and sweetener.
4. Add the eggs and vanilla extract to bowl and mix with an electric mixer for 1 minute until smooth.
5. Add melted chocolate and stir with a wooden spoon or spatula until the chocolate is incorporated into the butter mixture.
6. In a separate bowl, mix the dry ingredients (remaining ingredients besides walnuts) until combined.
7. Add dry ingredients into the bowl with the wet ingredients and stir with a wooden spoon until combined.

8. Add walnuts if desired.
9. Pour batter into prepared pan. Spread to cover the entire bottom of the pan and into corners.
10. Place in the center rack of the oven and bake for 30 minutes.
11. After the brownies are baked, take them out and leave them in the pan to cool.
12. When cool, cut them into 9 servings, and they are ready to eat.

These have to be a once-in-a-while treat because they are sweet, and if you're like me, that sugar will continue to call your name. These are so good you will have to work to eat only one serving.

Chocolate Chip Cookies

Chocolate cookies are a staple in most homes. You don't have to miss out just because you are on a low carbohydrate diet. These cookies will not be easily identifiable as low carb. That makes this a nice treat to share, so you aren't tempted to eat the entire batch.

Prep & Cooking Time: 30 mins

Servings: 24 cookies
Nutrition Facts: Calories: 120 | Carbohydrates: 3g | Protein: 2g | Fat: 11g

Ingredients:

1 ½ c almond flour
1 t baking powder
½ t salt
½ c butter, softened
½ c stevia
1 t vanilla extract
1 large egg
1 c sugar-free chocolate chips
½ c nuts, chopped

Instructions:

1. Preheat oven to 350 degrees.

2. Grease cookie sheets with butter and set aside.
3. In a large bowl, cream together the butter and the stevia.
4. Add the large egg and vanilla extract to the butter and stevia.
5. Mix until the egg is incorporated into the butter.
6. In a second bowl, mix together almond flour, baking powder, and salt until mixed well.
7. Add dry ingredients to the large bowl and mix until it is combined.
8. Add sugar-free chocolate chips and nuts and stir until they are distributed evenly.
9. Drop by spoonfuls onto the cookie sheet.
10. Bake until golden brown and the surface of cookies appear dry on the top and are cooked all the way through.
11. Remove cookies from sheet to a wire rack to cool.

Make these with or without nuts. Cocoa nibs can be used in place of the sugar-free chocolate chips. This is a good recipe to keep on hand so you can have a cookie along with everyone else. Make it a fun project with kids or friends. Baking is always a good way to bring people together, and this a recipe everyone will enjoy.

Keto Brown Butter Pralines

Quick and easy dessert with one net carb. Use a natural granulated sweetener like stevia to make the most of this recipe. There is some cooking, but no baking for these sweet tasty treats. Sprinkle with sea salt to add the salted caramel flavor that is so popular today.

Prep & Cooking Time: 16 mins

Servings: 10 servings
Nutrition Facts: Calories: 338 | Carbohydrates: 1g | Protein: 2g | Fat: 36g

Ingredients:

2 Sticks Salted butter
⅔ c heavy cream
⅔ c monk fruit sweetener
½ t xanthan gum
2 c pecans, chopped
Sea salt

Instructions:

1. Line a cookie sheet with parchment paper or use a silicone baking mat.
2. Prepare a cookie sheet with parchment paper or a silicone baking mat.

3. In a medium-size, medium weight saucepan, brown the butter until it smells nutty. Don't burn the butter. This will take about 5 minutes.
4. Stir in heavy cream, xanthan gum, and sweetener.
5. Take the pan off the heat and stir in the nuts.
6. Place pan in the refrigerator for an hour.
7. Stir the mixture occasionally while it is getting colder.
8. After an hour, scoop the mixture onto the cookie sheets and shape into cookies.
9. Sprinkle with sea salt.
10. Refrigerate on cookies sheet until the pralines are hard.
11. After the cookies are hard, transfer to an airtight container in the refrigerator.

This is a special treat. A low carb praline with the fat from the butter and cream. It is a nice dessert to have on a special occasion that you can work into your day without totally messing up your macros. The monk fruit sweetener is a 1:1 measure, so the texture is not altered by not using sugar. Give them a try and you will not be disappointed.

Conclusion

Thank you for making it through to the end of *Keto Diet for Women Over 50*, let's hope it was informative and able to provide you with all of the tools you need to achieve your goals in weight loss and a healthier lifestyle.

As women grow older, there are a variety of changes occurring within their bodies. Having a great deal of impact, the reduction of estrogen often causes weight gain and a slower metabolism. The keto diet, with adjustments for the particular requirements of women over fifty years old, is a wonderful way to lose weight while relieving some of the aches and pains experienced as the lack of estrogen takes hold. By adapting the diet to make it more palatable for women over the age of 50, the ketogenic diet can be beneficial in more ways than just weight loss. Follow the principals of food choices suggested by studies performed around the world and reap the benefits of this popular diet. Ease into ketosis with the plan outlined and you will find a smoother transition to a low-carbohydrate lifestyle. Use the tips and tricks given to smooth over rough spots and use the food list to try new foods.

You will have the most success on the keto diet by keeping track of your macros Maintain a record of the nutritional value of the foods you eat to avoid overeating. It can be easy to eat an excess of calories when putting an emphasis on eating fats. Eating a lot of meat makes it easy to eat an excess of protein. Failure to read labels can mean eating an unintended amount of carbohydrates. Take the time to learn what foods you like best and make plan your meals and snacks, so you stay on your macros. Make sure you eat lots of vegetable fiber and drink lots of water. The diet will work best when you to the time to count grams and calories.

You have the tools to be successful in losing weight on the keto diet. In the end, the weight loss will be the frosting on the. Don't worry; the cake will be made from almond flour and the frosting from stevia.

Finally, if you found this book useful in any way, a review on Amazon is always appreciated!

Made in the USA
Middletown, DE
08 December 2020